PILLAR ONE
STRESS LESS
SLEEP BETTER

The Busy Professional's Guide to Mastering Stress
& Achieving Perfect Sleep in Three Weeks

Re think

First published in Great Britain in 2021
by Rethink Press (www.rethinkpress.com)

© Copyright Riad Hechame

All rights reserved. No part of this publication may be reproduced, stored in or introduced into a retrieval system, or transmitted, in any form, or by any means (electronic, mechanical, photocopying, recording or otherwise) without the prior written permission of the publisher.

The right of Riad Hechame to be identified as the author of this work has been asserted by him in accordance with the Copyright, Designs and Patents Act 1988.

This book is sold subject to the condition that it shall not, by way of trade or otherwise, be lent, resold, hired out, or otherwise circulated without the publisher's prior consent in any form of binding or cover other than that in which it is published and without a similar condition including this condition being imposed on the subsequent purchaser.

Cover design courtesy of HELLO NASH.

Cover image © Adobe Stock / CLIPAREA

Praise

'This book is a wealth of techniques to allow you to master the basics of peak recovery: sleep and stress management. If you are in the fitness industry as a personal trainer or strength coach, this book will definitely give you a solid understanding on how to optimise your training/recovery ratio for training and performance results.'
— **Andre Benoit**, former Olympian in luge, world-renowned strength coach and owner of the Canadian Center for Strength and Conditioning (CCSC)

'Great book from one of the health and fitness industry's up-and-coming stars. Feeling the effects of stress? Under recovery? This book is for you. Riad expertly writes about different types of stress and the strategies to help combat them. This is a fantastic resource that I personally will come back to whenever I feel that my health could be suffering.'
— **Yas Parr**, strength and performance coach and published author

'For the past decade, sleep and recovery methods have been among the most studied variables in peaking human performance. This book will begin to bridge the gap between human performance and sleep recovery, providing extensive insight into the

emotional, developmental and longitudinal effects that sleep has on the human body.'
  — **Preston Green**, director of strength and conditioning, Florida Gators

'As a martial arts competitor for the past four decades, I quickly came to understand the importance of resting. It's not just about skipping a workout once in a while to allow your body to recover or dissipate the lactic acid from the previous workout, it's about shutting down your brain and recharging its batteries. There are all sorts of supplements and pills out there that could help you get a clearer view of things but the ONE true thing that really makes the difference and is a game changer is to simply have a good night sleep. Adopting a healthy sleeping pattern is the best way to recuperate and grow. *This book will teach you exactly that.* Now go on, have a good night of sleep.'
  — **Georges Galarregi**, devoted martial artist

'This book shares with you how to deal with different types of stress and how to improve the quality of your sleep. As a mother of a toddler, insufficient sleep is part of the job. More often than not, we tend to rush through the day dealing with different types of stress without realising that it affects how our day ends. Little did I know. How you respond to everything from the moment you wake up will dictate the quality of your sleep. This book may sound like it is for athletes, but even a non-athlete like me has picked up quite a few tips to improve the quality of my sleep. It has also reminded me that self-care is not just about taking care of my wellbeing, it is also about taking care of my sleep.'

— **Soo Fong**, lawyer and client

Disclaimer

The author has taken three years to write this book and undertake the related research with the greatest care. The content is based on information from sources he believes to be reliable, and he has made every reasonable effort to convey the information as completely and accurately as possible, but completeness and accuracy cannot be guaranteed.

The author offers the information in this book solely as a human-performance coach. Readers are strongly advised to consult with a physician, psychologist, psychiatrist or other licensed healthcare professional before utilising any of the information in this book.

*In memory of my adoptive mother Zeyneb,
who ingrained in me the love for detail and perfection.*

*And my mentor, Charles R Poliquin:
'My brain is wired for optimal, I don't like normal. I'm a
high-performance guy.'*

Contents

Foreword	1
Introduction	7
PART ONE One Week To Perfect Sleep	**19**
1 The Link Between Sleep And Health	21
Diving your way to great sleep	24
Do you know your chronotype?	26
Why eight doesn't equal eight	27
How much sleep do we really need?	28
2 What Bad Sleep Can Do To You	31
How our body is affected by bad sleep	31
How our mind is affected by bad sleep	35
How our health is affected by bad sleep	42
3 What Good Sleep Can Do For You	49
How our body recovers with good sleep	50
How our mind recovers with good sleep	51

How our health improves with good sleep	55
4 Techniques To Achieve Perfect Sleep In One Week – Quick Wins	**61**
Timing	62
Nutrition and supplements	67
Environment	70
Mind and body	73
Part One: Conclusion Perfect Sustainable Sleep	**81**
PART TWO Two Weeks to Master Stress	**85**
5 How Does Stress Affect Your Health?	**87**
Stress keeps you alive	88
How stress works	89
HPA axis	94
The cortisol dilemma	95
6 The Sources Of Stress	**99**
Genetic stress	100
Lifestyle stress	101
Social stress	101
Financial stress	102
Environmental stress	103
Nutritional stress	103
The emitter/receptor approach	104
The genotyping approach	105

7	**Mastering Genetic Stress – Immediate Wins**	**107**
	Ignore it	108
	Change your position or activity	109
	Fake it until you make it	110
	Sense when you need time	111
	Retreat	112
	Tune your heart in to coherence	112
	Power breathing	115
8	**Mastering Genetic Stress – Long-term Wins**	**121**
	Remain childlike	121
	Learn optimism	123
	Ask yourself if you're a stress inducer	124
	Never complain	125
	Be grateful and forgive	126
	Fight the right fight	129
	Sweet past, unknown present, scary future	129
	Change your perspective	131
	There are no problems, just challenges	131
	Master doing nothing	132
	Don't overthink things	133
	Use your imagination	134
	Your routine is your descendants' heritage	137
9	**Mastering Lifestyle Stress – Immediate Wins**	**139**
	First activity dictates your day	140
	Learn effective organisation	140

Put things back	141
Don't do to be, be to be	142
Learn proper prioritisation	143
Finish what you start	143
Avoid multitasking	144
Avoid accumulation	145
Be on time	146
Be cortisol friendly	146
Don't forget about breaks	147
Stop thinking about work during your free time	148
Don't buy stress	149
Your clothes	149
Learn to cook	150
You don't have to keep pace with your technology	151
Virtual detox	151
Choose your source of information wisely	154
Get a chauffeur	154
10 Mastering Lifestyle Stress – Long-term Wins	**157**
Embrace failure	157
Take care of yourself	159
Sense when you have got to take a break	159
Sense when to take a task by storm	160
Schedule work around holidays	161
Sport is a stressor	162

Overtraining	165
Be minimalistic	167
Don't swim against the flow	168
11 Mastering Social Stress – Immediate Wins	**171**
Smile	172
Greeting	173
Perception	174
Reconfirm	176
Be kind(er)	176
Give without expecting	177
Never compare yourself to others	177
Never promise	178
Power hug	179
Rely on nobody but yourself	180
Look for solutions not accusations	180
You don't have to convince	181
Mind love	181
Avoid being dependent	182
Avoid toxic people	182
Take time to judge	183
Honour your decisions	183
Don't ask for things you don't like to be asked for	184
12 Mastering Social Stress – Long-term Wins	**185**
Social circle and the solar system	185
Build your tribe	186

Have brothers and sisters	186
Children	187
Your kids' stress	190
Be yourself	194
Care less about others' opinions	194
Contact with officials	196
Colleagues and lakes	196
Invest in good relationships	197
Don't speak negatively of others	197
Don't spread the bad word	198
Reveal no more than necessary	199
Judge situations, not people	199
13 Mastering Financial Stress	**201**
Don't be extravagant	202
Lead by love and example	203
Progress and grow	204
Work on the weak link	205
Build an independent business	206
Build a business you love	207
Passive and active staff	208
Price doesn't always equal value	209
Define your required value of a thing prior to purchase	209
Your ability to make money is more important than money	211

14 Managing Environmental Stress — 215

- Information abstention — 216
- Mind unnecessary sounds — 216
- Eat naturally — 217
- Extreme temperatures — 218
- Don't fear complexity — 219
- Your space — 220
- Go back to nature — 221
- Be rough — 221
- Smart use of smart devices — 223
- Junk light — 224
- Mind toxins — 226
- Detoxify — 229
- Beware of mould — 232

15 Mastering Nutritional Stress — 237

- Gut rebuilding — 240
- You need more fat than sugar — 241
- Watch your meal frequency — 242
- Eat only when the sun is out — 242
- Your morning friend becomes your evening enemy — 243
- Divorce from allergens — 243
- Take care of your friends — 244
- What you like may not like you — 245
- Clean up your kitchen — 245

Fasting	246
Lifestyle versus dieting	246
Conclusion	**249**
Acknowledgements	**253**
The Author	**255**

Foreword

Would you say that you are at your peak performance level mentally and physically when you are sick, have a fever, cough every few minutes, have an upset stomach? It seems easy to answer: 'No, of course not' without a second thought, but what if you don't have any of these symptoms? Are you at your peak then? Is 'not being sick' a good indication of recovery?

Life passes by at the speed of light and we live in an era where performance is a must: we need to set and meet goals, and achieve optimal results not only at work, but in our personal lives as well. Nowadays, it seems that we even need to perform during our time off. Relaxing is not just relaxing anymore; it's meditating, and being good at it too. To top it off, we are living in the days of the binary way of thinking (right/wrong, yes/no, good/bad, start/finish). Actions we take to attain peak performance are either good or bad, helping or counteracting. There is no grey area or time to adapt and reflect. Staying focused on your goal *is* the goal.

It's easy to look online, on TV, in books or podcasts to find cure-it-all methods to increase performance. I've been in the health and fitness industry for over twenty-eight years and I've seen plenty of revolutionary concepts come and go. One thing I know for sure: it is impossible to always have more things to do and endlessly achieve peak performance on all fronts. That's the best recipe for burning the candle at both ends.

One area of performance that is too often underestimated is recovery and its most important component, sleep. Cutting down on sleep to achieve more may seem like a good idea – surely it would give you more time to do more things? Or you may think that your sleeping habits are already good, but are you aware that the quality of your sleep can be a barrier to your level of achievement?

The evaluation of the quality of sleep is highly subjective simply because we are unconscious when we are sleeping. We can only rely on how we feel when we wake up in the morning and if we were awake or not during the night. Unfortunately, both markers are inaccurate.

FOREWORD

In a study by Dr William Dement, an American sleep researcher and founder of the Sleep Research Center at Stanford University, participants were allowed to sleep for only 2 hours (from 5am to 7am).[1] They were then asked to sit at a computer for an hour and note every 2 minutes how likely they were to fall asleep in the next 2 minutes. The results: participants fell asleep many times when they had evaluated their chances at 0%, and then stayed awake in moments when they'd scored themselves at 100% likely to fall asleep. Moreover, the sleep episodes lasted for 3 seconds or more without them being aware of having slept at all. Three seconds may not seem major, but if you are operating machinery or driving at 100 km/h during that short period of time, results could be fatal.

Numerous studies have shown that we can have micro cycles of sleep without noticing it. Airplane pilots were monitored (brainwave recorded) before landing after an overnight eight-hour flight.[2] Even if the pilots knew they were being monitored with researchers around them, and were fighting to show how well they were staying awake and alert, they had moments of sleep with their eyes open (periods of 1 to 20 seconds). The truth is they didn't notice they were sleeping (which makes sense if they were unconscious). If

---

1 William Dement, W Dement and C Vaughan, *The Promise of Sleep* (2000), Dell
2 N Wright and A McGown, 'Vigilance on the civil flight deck: incidence of sleepiness and sleep during long-haul flights and associated changes in physiological parameters' (2001), www.ncbi.nlm.nih.gov/pubmed/11214900

we as humans are unable to evaluate such small episodes, how can we be good at evaluating a full night's sleep?

Pushing endlessly to perform without proper recovery is like pressing on the button to call an elevator twenty times in a row, hoping it will make it arrive faster, or pushing harder on the TV remote control when its battery levels are low to change the channels. An on/off switch can't be influenced by different pressure or several hits. No matter how frequently or how hard your press, it won't accelerate the process.

The same applies to your performance. Always pushing harder is not the best way to achieve your goal. Often, simply recharging your batteries may be the best option, and it is valid for everyone. I have worked with top-level athletes for whom recovery is mandatory before a major competition. It's part of the planning to taper down the intensity in the gym while optimising their performance.

Since we can't be good judges of the quality of our sleep, we need to assume that it can only be improved and that our recovery may not currently be optimal. That is what this book is all about: addressing every aspect of our sleep routine, allowing us to reduce stress by improving our psychological state, and finally achieving peak recovery.

FOREWORD

I first met Riad when he flew in from Hong Kong for an internship with me in Montreal, Canada. Talk about motivation and dedication – he'd surely had to test his knowledge of the principles of recovery on himself. As a full-time engineer designing and commissioning nuclear power plants, married with four kids, owner of a successful fitness-coaching business, studying in the health and fitness fields, constantly travelling around the globe to learn from his mentors, working on the construction of his new strength and performance clinic in Kuala Lumpur while living in Hong Kong and remaining successful in each and every one of these areas, he would not have found this possible without proper recovery. On top of that, add the three years of time and energy Riad spent working on this book.

In *Stress Less, Sleep Better*, you'll find techniques to optimise recovery, how to get better sleep, quality and quantity, what supplements could be helpful, etc. But what strikes me most is how Riad is able to step aside from science and show his vulnerability by sharing his personal philosophy of life.

Stay hungry for your goals and *Stress Less, Sleep Better*.

Christian Maurice, certified functional medicine practitioner, lecturer and owner of Elemental World (www.ElementalWorld.com)

Introduction

It only takes three steps to glory.

Since human life began on earth, competition has been a main driver for increasing our performance. We've continually strived to be stronger, sprint faster, jump higher, throw further etc. It's part of our instinct for survival. In the past, anyone who couldn't keep their performance at a high level risked being sacrificed first in wars, dying from hunger or ending up as a predator's meal.

When the lightbulb was invented, we began spending more and more time working indoors. Our survival was secured through employment and suddenly there was no real need to have the skills our ancestors had. With the advent of the electronic age, we've taken an even more extreme step towards the sedentary life. Much of the need for human-power has been replaced by more efficient, reliable and cost-saving robotics.

Of course, not all segments of society lead a sedentary lifestyle. Athletes, for example, continue to work on their physical performance to this day. But what about the performance of others? Do we need to be at a peak of physical fitness even if we are just using our fingertips? We still need to be able to use our brains and remember experiences, numbers, analyse data, make the right decisions etc, so are our intellectual and smart abilities exempt from measurement on a performance scale?

What office warriors and academics have in common with professional high-level athletes is goal setting. We all have specific goals that we are striving for, but what differentiates us is that athletes are already at their peak of performance. They have learned to optimise every aspect in their lives, from recovery to nutrition and training. Even if they get injured or have surgery, they know how to rehabilitate fast and continue climbing to peak again within a short time.

Why can't this happen for everyone? Why are some of us so far away from our peak performance? My personal view on this question is that we can be too focused on the target itself, while neglecting everything else. Busy producing results, we can forget about basic elements like sleep, stress management,

INTRODUCTION

nutrition and exercise. There are many people who truly believe they don't have enough time for those things, so they cut down on sleep, eat on the go and feel there's no need to talk about exercising.

Do you imagine you can be anywhere near your personal peak performance if you are:

- Sleeping fewer than 8 hours per night?
- Consulting your mobile phone 200+ times per day, using it directly prior to going to sleep and as an alarm clock to wake you up, living in an electromagnetic field (EMF) cloud surrounded by displays and blue-light emitters?
- Not taking care of your state of mind?
- Eating pro-inflammatory foods, genetically modified organisms (GMOs) and foods loaded with pesticides?
- Abstaining from eating essential proteins and fats?
- Abstaining from high-quality supplementation to bridge the gap?
- Not exercising at all or doing a load of stress-inducing high-volume cardio?

Here's the bitter truth enrobed in a sweet cover: you have plenty of potential. I'm going to teach you the three pillars of human performance: recovery, nutrition and training. When correctly constructed and maintained, these three pillars will take you to your highest level of fitness, wellbeing and happiness. In this book, we're going to focus on pillar one: recovery – because a well-recovered body can become a fit body. We'll look at the two major limiting factors that all busy professionals face: lack of sleep and overload of stress.

When you know how to get the perfect night's sleep and wake feeling refreshed and rejuvenated, you will be able to face the world with confidence and vigour. Understanding stress, how to manage and mitigate it, you'll be in control of the way you react to the world. When you take control of stress and get the perfect night's sleep, your physical training will progress quickly, you'll recover more easily from injury or overwork, you'll build muscle and you'll achieve your peak performance.

In this book, I will provide tools and techniques you can start using immediately, then I'll give you ongoing methodologies to make sure you control your stress and achieve perfect sleep in the long term. This is not a quick-fix guide – this is your lifetime blueprint for sustained peak recovery. Pick a couple of techniques that resonate most with you or are easy to implement and apply them step by step. Once they become part of your lifestyle, when you don't have to think about doing them anymore, pick your next techniques and do the same. Once you have established a

INTRODUCTION

robust circadian rhythm with high-quality sleep, do the same with Part Two, Two Weeks To Master Stress.

As with everything in life, the methodologies I share in this book are not black and white, so the transition from one chapter, section or technique to the next is not necessarily linear. Once you master one technique, you can move on to the next, but listen to your instincts. This journey is a personal challenge so you need to understand your instincts if you wish to be successful.

You won't actually need to implement all of the techniques listed in this book, but you will massively benefit by implementing the techniques which are the most suitable to your personality type. You will find techniques which you already apply naturally and don't even have to think about, because they are in line with your personality type or genotype. You will also find techniques which seem unnatural or hard to implement. Those are normally the ones you will benefit the most from by following step by step.

I can't take full credit for all the techniques I'll discuss in this book. As the adage goes, we don't need to reinvent the wheel. Rather I have adapted and optimised tried-and-tested techniques to achieve peak performance. To build peak human performance, we need a blueprint; a guide; some instructions. Every construction has pillars, and in my world, as a strength and human-performance coach, there are three:

1. Recovery – recover like a baby
2. Nutrition – eat like a predator
3. Training – train like a gladiator

These three pillars are not only the base for peak performance but also the fundamentals for healthy aging by protecting our DNA against damage. Nobel Prize winning scientist Dr Elizabeth Blackburn and health psychologist Dr Elissa Epel showed that in overstressed people their telomeres, which are the protective caps at the end of our chromosomes and responsible for how fast we age, stopped the rapid shortening once sleep and nutrition were fixed. The amazing thing is, once exercising was added to the routine of those persons, their telomeres started regenerating and getting longer which is equivalent to reversed aging.[3]

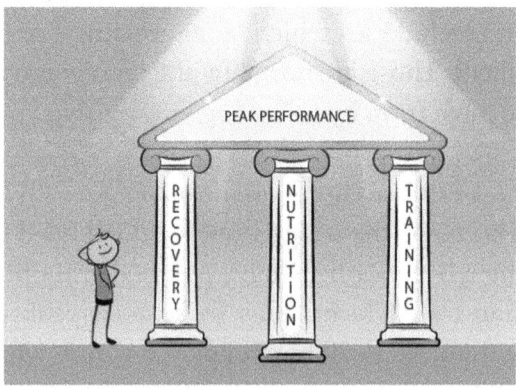

---

3   Eli Puterman et al., 'Determinants of telomere attrition over one year in healthy older women: Stress and health behaviors matter' (2014), www.ncbi.nlm.nih.gov/pmc/articles/PMC4310821

INTRODUCTION

The first pillar to achieving peak human performance, *recovery*, will allow you to establish complete harmony in your circadian rhythm (recurring naturally every 24 hours) by increasing your quality and quantity of sleep. The next target is to teach you the different sources of stress and how you can be in control of each one of them, depending on your character type. You will be able to quickly establish a positive balance between your stress levels and your recovery, increasing your capacity to handle stress and recover fast. The third target is the use of meditation to find harmony between yourself and the universe.

With these three main targets to achieving peak recovery, you will be able to completely shut down and reenergise after a stressful day, a hard workout or both, and start the next day with body and mind fully recovered and tuned to tackle new challenges.

The second pillar to achieving peak human performance is *nutrition*.[4] Besides teaching you to eat healthily and apply the right meal frequency and macronutrient mix according to your genetics, peak nutrition has these main targets:

- Helping you fight against excessive inflammation
- Helping you restore your gut flora and reestablish your gut lining

---

4   *Eat Better, Feel Greater* is the second pillar in this series.

- Supporting your main detoxification organs to work properly
- Boosting your immune system
- Healing your brain to achieve peak cognitive function with the ability to retain information and learn more

We will cover advanced nutritional methodologies, which go hand in hand with the training methodologies in *Pillar Three*[5], to help you achieve fast results by alternating optimal physical growth with phases of fasting or caloric restriction for fat loss, mental growth, self-discipline, rejuvenation and detoxification.

The last pillar is all about losing body fat, improving your body composition, being strong and achieving peak physical and mental performance. The main focus here is to help you to find a healthy progression in strength and performance until you reach your peak levels. We will work on your mobility, movement functionality, structural balance and posture, focusing on continuously increasing your strength levels, helping you increase your work capacity and build muscle mass, even if your workplace is the office.

Once you have achieved a performance-friendly lifestyle by building a strong base on the three pillars, the sky will be your limit. Your brain will be fast-acting and deep-thinking with strong visualisation capabili-

---

5   *Get Stronger, Become Younger* is the third pillar of this series.

ties all set up to pursue new challenges. You'll find self-confidence, motivation and optimal strength, and take on new ideas and challenges with interest and respect rather than fear and anxiety, seeing in them potential opportunities to progress and grow.

This base will help you unleash your potential and break any limitations you may have set for yourself, but more importantly, it will send a message from your brain that your body needs all of your organs working properly in tandem with your muscle mass, bone density, posture etc. Enabling your body to work at peak performance regularly is the best natural anti-aging process available. That's what peak recovery, nutrition and training are about. It's nothing magical, but the results are certainly wonderful.

This book is specific to the first pillar, *peak recovery*, and focuses on *sleep* and *stress*. We will touch on the science behind each and dive into specific techniques to master both. In the following books, we will address EMF stress, meditation and advanced techniques for stress management.

I once asked my mentor and friend, Charles R Poliquin, what his advice would be for his twenty-year-old self. His answer was:

> 'Increase sleep time and reduce work hours. I was sleeping just a couple of hours and working 18 hours a day'.

Charles is the most successful strength and performance coach who ever lived, if measured by Olympic medallists and world record holders. Once this rule was applied to his new company, within a few months he was making more money from one individual than from a team of thirty at his former company.

HARD RECOVERY PRECEDES HARD WORK, AND HARD WORK PRECEDES HARD WINS

Proper recovery is the main pillar to achieving peak performance. Trying to be useful without proper recovery from the daily activities is like trying to erect a building without foundations. The building will collapse sooner or later under its own weight, but this fundamental attribute is by far the most neglected, especially by those who want to become peak performers.

There is no point in thinking about proper nutrition, supplementation and training if you are messing with your recovery. There are no vitamins, protein shakes or methodologies which can help you do better if your recovery is compromised.

In this book, we will discuss the principal tools of recovery you have to have in your toolbox if you are serious about your peak performance. Sleep is the main one, followed by stress management. In the following book, we will dive into the second approach to managing stress, the genotyping approach, exploring advanced methodologies and the wonderful world of science-based meditation.

In Part One of this book, we will discuss sleep and its importance to the human body in detail. Then I'll present to you a collection of practical techniques to prepare yourself for uninterrupted, deep and good-quality sleep to recharge your body and brain. In Part Two, we will discuss the emitter/receptor approach – the first approach to stress management – diving into different methodologies to build a strong castle, so to speak, in a friendly environment.

Let's get started!

PART ONE
ONE WEEK TO PERFECT SLEEP

Focus on sleep and all the rest will fall in place.

1
The Link Between Sleep And Health

You can't fully experience wakefulness during the day if your sleep during the night is compromised.

Everyone is likely to know about the importance of sleep, but too often we forget the crucial link between sleep, both good and bad, and our health. In this part, we will address sleep as being the backbone of enhancing recovery, reducing stress and empowering not only rejuvenation and anti-aging, but also mental and physical performance.

After looking at a few introductory principles of sleep, we will dive into the major health implications of bad sleep and the diseases it can generate. We will then turn to the benefits good-quality sleep has on both health and performance. I will present simple techniques to enjoying rejuvenating sleep in record time, then we'll discuss broadly used hacks to fix sleep that you should avoid and how to implement techniques for sustainable results in the long term.

There are three main links between sleep and health:

1. **Sleep is the most important solution for stress management.** This is the main fundamental to achieving your peak performance and without it you won't even get close. Trying to manage stress without proper sleep would be like driving a car with flat tyres. Your performance will be compromised and risk of doing damage is high. Proper sleep is not a luxury, but rather an absolute necessity.

2. **During sleep, you recover from the day before.** If your sleep quality and quantity are poor, you will not fully recover and fatigue will accumulate from day to day until you reach a state of chronic fatigue. The big negative impact will not only be on your performance, but more importantly on your health.

3. **During sleep you detoxify.** You regenerate and build new cells, including neurons, release growth hormones (GHs) and other androgens, and produce neurotransmitters. Sleep is the antidote to fear and anxiety, aging and degenerative diseases. If your brain were a computer, you

could view sleep as the mechanism to reboot your system and reset the memory.

I have always been amazed by how many people naively think that a few hours of sleep will be enough and question why they should waste time sleeping if they could accomplish more things otherwise. I'm not being extreme in saying this; I've heard it many times. People can become so focused on the main goal of increasing their performance, they ignore the fact that every peak must have a base and a foundation.

Good-quality sleep is fundamental to good health, wellbeing and the quality of work, achievements and performance.

I once had a conversation with a highly ranked colleague. She was talking about her techniques to be more productive, and when I asked her what her trick was, hoping to learn something new, she said with conviction that she was sleeping less. She had taught herself that she just needed a maximum of 4 hours' sleep per night because she had more important tasks and responsibilities to manage, and she was feeling 'splendid'.

Seven years later, I had a conversation along the same lines with another high-ranking colleague. His answer was similar: he had cut down on his sleep time to be able to achieve more, but he recognised that his strategy had failed as he was abusing and disrespecting his body.

This second example showed me where this particular way of saving time can lead. My colleague was literally falling apart. He was overstressed, having problems with stomach pains, suffering from sleeping disorders and an atrophied torso, and was weak in general. He was also having difficulties concentrating and recalling important information. Tasks he had once been brilliant at, such as memorising any type of information and doing complex maths calculations in his mind, were now causing him problems. And, most disturbingly of all, he was still under thirty years of age. He recognised the necessity for change and asked me to coach him.

Diving your way to great sleep

Sleep may seem like a passive time where we close shop and reopen the next day, but it's not a homogeneous state, and that's especially true for the brain. When we fall asleep, we go through multiple consecutive cycles, each of which lasts for about 90 minutes.

When we dive into a sleep cycle, we start with the shallow sleep, which is called rapid eye movement (REM). We continue to dive deeper until we hit the non-rapid eye movement (NREM) with its different stages, which depend on sleep depth.

THE LINK BETWEEN SLEEP AND HEALTH

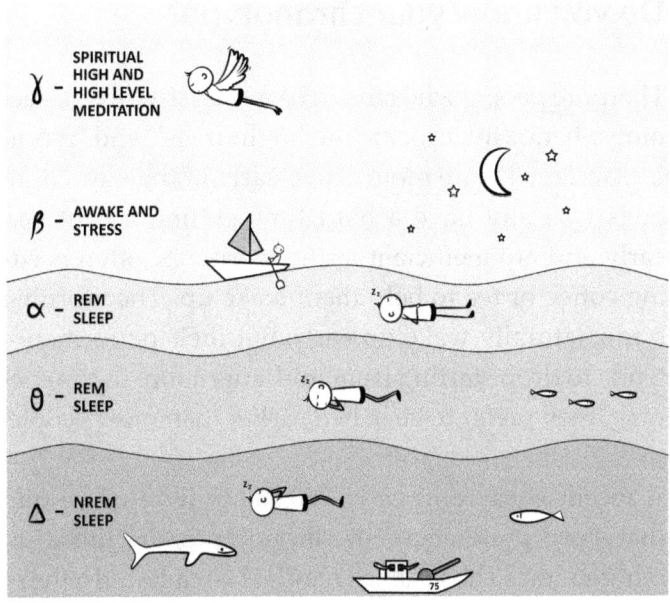

Each phase has its corresponding processes, which are also consecutively scheduled. During NREM sleep, neurons are firing in their slowest pattern – delta brainwaves with their cleansing powers – and the information in the short-term memory is being copied into the part of the brain where long-term memory is stored. During REM sleep, healing and rejuvenating alpha brainwaves are being emitted and the brain interconnects all the pieces of information with each other. It's during the REM sleep that our emotional quotient (EQ) is fostered.[6]

---

6   Matthew Walker, *Why we sleep: the new science of sleep and dreams* (Penguin, 2007).

Do you know your chronotype?

There are people who tend to be more active in the evenings, hence their nickname 'night owls', and 'morning birds' who are more active early in the day. Night owls typically have a hard time getting out of bed early and are inefficient in the mornings, often needing coffee or tea to help them wake up. The morning birds naturally wake up early, but their performance tends to drop starting from mid-afternoon. In the evening, they prefer to be in bed earlier than most people.

A recent study on nearly 700,000 individuals found that sleep preferences, or chronotypes, are linked to our genome. Those genes regulate circadian rhythms. The same study found that people with the early riser chronotype are happier and less likely to have depression or mental health issues.[7]

On one hand, our genetic makeup may express itself in us being a night owl or morning bird, but we also have our epigenetics, which are heavily influenced by our behaviours and the decisions we make in life. As our occupation and external stimuli, such as environmental light levels and temperature, impact on our chronotype and may shift it in one direction or another, we can also take the correct action to shift our chronotype towards the golden sleep window of

---

7   S E Jones, J M Lane and M N Weedon, 'Genome-wide association analyses of chronotype in 697,828 individuals provides insights into circadian rhythms' (2019), www.nature.com/articles/s41467-018-08259-7

10pm to 6am as long as we have a job that makes this possible. I have seen evidence of this from my own experience and that of clients whom I have helped to shift to this window in a short timeframe.

Why eight doesn't equal eight

Opinions may differ on the best timespan for sleep. Personally, I need to be asleep no later than 10pm if I really want to be at my peak the next day. Just half an hour later and I definitely feel the drawbacks during the day with less energy and clarity of thought.

The positive effects during early sleep are profound. An hour between 10pm and 11pm doesn't equate to an hour between 6am and 7am. It's not possible to gain the benefits of early sleep once you've missed the best sleeping time as sleep is not a homogenous state of the brain. During the early hours, we are more in deep NREM sleep, and later on we have more REM and light NREM sleep. The early hours of sleep are crucially important for memory saving.

A further argument in favour of going to bed early is that you avoid the typical binge time in the kitchen. Feedback and experience have shown me that the late evening hours are when people tend to struggle the most to resist carbs. By going to bed early, you eradicate the risk of temptation and increase your chances of getting into shape in record time.

How much sleep do we really need?

Research has shown that the safe window of sleep for adults is between 7 and 9 hours, but there is evidence that 8 hours of sleep is the golden number.[8] After 10 days of sleeping 6 hours, the brain is as dysfunctional as if you'd missed one whole night's sleep.

A recent sleep extension study suggests that the average underlying sleep tendency in young adults is about 8.5 hours per night. By comparison, the average reported sleep length of 7.2–7.4 hours is deficient, and common sleep length of 6.5 hours or under can be disastrous.[9]

Fewer than 6.5 or more than 9.5 hours is potentially harmful. Certainly, there are people who come out just fine under these circumstances, but they are rare cases. Ideally, sleep time needs to be somewhere between 8 and 8.5 hours. Furthermore, it has also been shown that a missed hour of sleep requires four proper night's sleep to recover from and not just one, as many of us think.[10]

---

8 J-P Chaput, C Dutil and H Sampasa-Kanyinga, 'Sleeping hours: what is the ideal number and how does age impact this?' (2018), www.ncbi.nlm.nih.gov/pmc/articles/PMC6267703/
9 M Bonnet et al., 'We are chronically sleep deprived' (1995), www.researchgate.net/publication/14456961_We_are_Chronically_Sleep_Deprived
10 S Kitamura et al., 'Estimating individual optimal sleep duration and potential sleep debt' (2016), www.ncbi.nlm.nih.gov/pmc/articles/PMC5075948/

Find out what works best for you. Check how you feel if you keep all parameters unchanged except for sleep duration and determine which length of time is optimal for you. You can also go to www.phpstrengthclinic.com/sleep and identify what the weakest links of your sleep are and what improvements you might need to achieve a better quality sleep.

If you are dead serious about your health and performance, your first concern must be fixing your sleep. Over the next couple of chapters, we will look at some arguments against bad sleep and for promoting good sleep, just in case you are still not convinced.

2
What Bad Sleep Can Do To You

Don't let sickness be your motivator.

Beside speeding up the aging process and having major implications on our physical and mental performance, not enough, interrupted or bad-quality sleep can promote major diseases such as cancer, diabetes and Alzheimer's. In this chapter, we will discuss recent scientific research on these implications and look at a case study on how prolonged periods of poor-quality sleep can manifest.

How our body is affected by bad sleep

Bad sleep has direct and deep impacts on the organism that is our body. It can negatively influence DNA repair, increase fat gain and muscle loss, be detrimental to the health of our microbiome and make us more prone to injuries or accidents.

Let's take a closer look at some of the negative effects on our body of not getting enough good-quality sleep.

Muscle atrophy. The combination of inadequate sleep and calorie-restricted diets (as is often the case during a weight-loss endeavour) will lead to muscle loss instead of fat loss. A study was undertaken on a group of overweight males and females who lived in a sleep research centre for two separate periods, lasting two weeks each.[11] During each period, they were on identical low-calorie diets, but during the first 2-week period, they had 8.5 hours sleep each night, while in the second period they slept for just 5.5 hours each night. They all lost about 7 lb during both periods, but they lost mainly muscle rather than fat during their sleep-deprived period.

Sleep deprivation increases catabolic hormone levels, favouring muscle protein breakdown and decreased androgen levels, which can counteract muscle protein synthesis. This will lead to catabolising of lean muscle

---

11 A V Nedeltcheva et al., 'Insufficient sleep undermines dietary efforts to reduce adiposity' (2010), https://annals.org/aim/article-abstract/746184/insufficient-sleep-undermines-dietary-efforts-reduce-adiposity

mass to fuel the everlasting fight-or-flight situation.[12][13] In other words, if your goal is a health transformation in which you target fat loss and muscle gain, then your first step should be fixing your sleep prior to implementing any dietary changes with calorie restriction.

Athletic performance and injury risk. Bad-quality or not enough sleep has a direct impact on athletic performance. Performance markers like speed and endurance, neurocognitive function – eg attention and memory – and physical health – eg mitigating illness and injury risk and maintaining weight – have all been shown to be negatively affected by insufficient sleep.[14] One major parameter which changes is the reduced time it takes to reach exhaustion.[15] After physical effort, lactic acid builds up quickly within the muscles, blood is poorly saturated in oxygen and carbon dioxide in the blood is high.

The impact of bad sleep on neurocognitive functions, such as attention and memory, also applies to the general population. If our sleep is compromised, then our overall performance suffers as well.

---

12 M Dattilo et al., 'Sleep and muscle recovery: endocrinological and molecular basis for a new and promising hypothesis' (2011), www.ncbi.nlm.nih.gov/pubmed/21550729
13 University of Chicago Medical Center, 'Sleep loss dramatically lowers testosterone in healthy young men' (2011), www.sciencedaily.com/releases/2011/05/110531162142.htm
14 N S Simpson et al., 'Optimizing sleep to maximize performance: implications and recommendations for elite athletes' (2017), www.ncbi.nlm.nih.gov/pubmed/27367265
15 T Van Helder et al., 'Sleep deprivation and the effect on exercise performance' (1989), www.ncbi.nlm.nih.gov/pubmed/2657963

Altered microbiome. Recent research has shown a clear link between sleep and microbiome health. Partial sleep deprivation alters the human gut microbiome, which has a direct impact on our cognitive function, stress and anxiety. Better sleep quality is associated with better cognitive function and higher proportions of gut microbial environment.[16]

Major neurotransmitters are produced in the gut by good bacteria. An unhealthy gut flora will have a direct impact on our neurotransmitter profile, which influences our drive, motivation and happiness.

DNA damage. In 2019, a study was undertaken on forty-nine healthy on-call doctors who were required to work overnight. They were found to have lower DNA repair gene expression and more DNA breaks than participants who did not work overnight.

Damaged DNA increases after only one night of sleep deprivation.[17] Because of DNA being the blueprint for the synthesis of the proteins our cells need to function, mutations can cause serious health issues, including the generation of cancerous cells.

16　J R Anderson et al., (2017), 'A preliminary examination of gut microbiota, sleep, and cognitive flexibility in healthy older adults' (2017), www.ncbi.nlm.nih.gov/pubmed/29031742

17　Wiley Newsroom, 'Sleep deprivation may affect our genes' (2019), https://newsroom.wiley.com/press-release/sleep-deprivation-may-affect-our-genes

Injury and accidents. Let's just focus here on accidents that happen when a car driver is drowsy rather than those that happen when people are sleep deprived while operating heavy machinery, such as flying a jet, or performing precision tasks, such as surgery. Yearly, there are thousands of victims of fatal accidents due to people driving while sleep deprived. Having fewer than 6 hours sleep in the previous 24 hours is associated with a six-fold increase in the odds of suffering from crash-related injuries.[18]

The 2009 Massachusetts Special Commission on Drowsy Driving estimated that there could be as many as 1.2 million crashes, 8,000 lives lost and 500,000 injuries each year attributed to people driving while overtired in the United States alone.[19] Sleep deprivation can lead to accidents in exactly the same way as drinking alcohol.

How our mind is affected by bad sleep

The impact of impaired sleep is not only limited to our bodies, it also has a huge impact on our minds. Bad sleep lowers our intelligence quotient (IQ), our EQ and our ability to forget negative experiences, which is an instinctive behaviour to survive and start a new

---

18 S Ameratunga et al., 'Driver sleepiness and risk of motor vehicle crash injuries: a population-based case control study in Fiji' (2014), www.ncbi.nlm.nih.gov/pubmed/23830198
19 National Highway Traffic Safety Administration, 'Drowsy driving' (2017), www.nhtsa.gov/risky-driving/drowsy-driving

day with positive thoughts. It reduces our capacity to tolerate stress and increases depression, anxiety, aggressive mood swings and possibly even suicidal thoughts.

Lower IQ. Getting less sleep than the recommended amount can cause an apparent IQ loss of five to eight points the next day, and population norm studies have shown that losing an entire night's sleep can lead to up to one standard deviation loss on our IQ.[20] In other words, we're effectively operating with the equivalent of a learning disability.

Lower EQ. During REM sleep cycles, our EQ and the interconnectivity between the different parts of the brain are fostered. Cutting the night's sleep results in fewer cycles of REM sleep, leading to an adverse impact on brain interconnectivity and lowered emotional intelligence and empathy. In other words, sleep deprivation, in a similar way to excessive mobile phone use, makes us less human.[21]

Atrophied brain. Recent research has shown that sleeping for too short a time (fewer than 6 hours) and too long a time (more than 9 hours) can lead to an

---

20 Tara Swart, 'Sleeping your way to the top' (2016), https://executive.mit.edu/blog/sleeping-your-way-to-the-top
21 C D Wiesner et al., 'The effect of selective REM-sleep deprivation on the consolidation and affective evaluation of emotional memories' (2015), www.ncbi.nlm.nih.gov/pubmed/25708092

atrophied total cerebral brain volume.[22] It's obvious that brain atrophy, in a similar way to muscle atrophy which is linked to loss in strength, endurance, bone density etc, is a bad thing. Brain atrophy is linked to memory loss, learning and attention deficit, an overall lowering of brain performance, such as trouble speaking or understanding, and even a loss of consciousness.

Dementia and Alzheimer's. Sleep deprivation of just one night (31 hours without sleep) has been shown to significantly increase the build-up of β-Amyloid protein in the right hippocampus and thalamus.[23] β-Amyloid protein, which is a metabolic waste product of neurons, is linked to dementia and Alzheimer's disease. This increase of β-Amyloid is also associated with mood worsening.

If our sleep quality and quantity are regularly compromised, then β-Amyloid protein and other waste products will build up as the natural detoxification process won't have enough time to rinse out all the metabolites. With enough build up, this could directly lead to dementia and Alzheimer's disease.

---

22 Andrew J Westwood et al., 'Prolonged sleep duration as a marker of early neurodegeneration predicting incident dementia' (2017), https://n.neurology.org/content/88/12/1172
23 Ehsan Shokri-Kojori et al., 'β-Amyloid accumulation in the human brain after one night of sleep deprivation' (2018), www.ncbi.nlm.nih.gov/pmc/articles/PMC5924922

High suicide risk. Increasing evidence suggests that disturbances in sleep are associated with an elevated risk of suicidal behaviours.[24] Both sleep disorders and general sleep complaints appear to be risk factors. In consideration of these findings, sleep problems and, more specifically, significant changes in sleep habits are now listed among the twelve warning signs of suicide from the Substance Abuse and Mental Health Services Administration.[25]

Often people ignore this risk and think they are mentally strong enough not to fall into this trap, but many studies have proven the association between bad sleep and high suicidal risk. What's also interesting is that these studies show that being less inclined towards depression has no moderating effect on the association. In other words, no one is safe from a high risk of suicidal thoughts when their sleep is compromised.

Reduced memory. During NREM sleep cycles, the brain moves the information it's stored in the short-term memory to the long-term memory, where it is safer. Reducing the quality and/or quantity of night sleep results in fewer cycles of NREM, resulting in a higher risk of memory loss.

---

24 Michael L Perlis et al., 'Suicide and sleep: Is it a bad thing to be awake when reason sleeps?' (2015), www.ncbi.nlm.nih.gov/pmc/articles/PMC5070474/
25 https://store.samhsa.gov/product/In-Brief-Substance-Use-and-Suicide-/sma16-4935

This has been shown in a study where a single night of sleep deprivation produced a significant deficit in hippocampal activity, the hippocampus being the region of the brain responsible for memory consolidation, and during memory encoding, resulting in a subsequent worsening of information retention.[26] If you have learned something new today, take special care of your sleep tonight and for the next few nights to consolidate the new information into your long-term memory. People with compromised sleep are more forgetful.

Impaired ability to forget negative experiences. Sleep plays a major role in the consolidation of memory, including emotional events, positive as well as negative, which the brain usually remembers better than neutral ones. A study has shown that while memories of neutral and positive events deteriorate after sleep deprivation, the ability to recall negative events remains the same.[27] In other words, with sleep deprivation, we're more likely to forget positive and neutral stimuli, while remembering bad experiences.

Impaired cognitive function. Sleep deprivation reduces regional cerebral metabolism within the prefrontal cortex, the region of the brain mostly responsible for higher-order cognitive processes, including

---

26 S S Yoo et al., 'A deficit in the ability to form new human memories without sleep' (2007), www.ncbi.nlm.nih.gov/pubmed/17293859/
27 Virginie Sterpenich et al., 'Sleep related Hippocampo-Cortical interplay during emotional memory recollection' (2007), www.ncbi.nlm.nih.gov/pmc/articles/PMC2039770/

judgment and decision making. Sleep deprived, we tend to make riskier decisions than usual. This vulnerability may become more pronounced with increased age.[28]

Sleep deprivation of just 17–19 hours renders our performance equivalent to or worse than that of someone with a blood alcohol content (BAC) of 0.05%, our reflexes being 50% slower than normal. After 28 hours without sleep, we are at an alcohol intoxication level of 0.1%.[29]

A recent laboratory study indicated that nocturnal sleep periods reduced by as little as 1.3 to 1.5 hours for one night resulted in a reduction of daytime alertness by as much as 32%.[30] If your work requires decision making and high alertness, you have to be careful with your sleep to improve your cognitive function and mental performance.

Stress tolerance. Sleep deprivation is a double-edged sword. Our sensing of stress goes up, which means the smallest stress input may induce a disproportionately strong reaction. We become less patient and get

---

28 W D Killgore, T J Balkin and N J Wesensten, 'Impaired decision making following 49 h of sleep deprivation' (2006), www.ncbi.nlm.nih.gov/pubmed/16489997
29 A M Williamson and A M Feyer 'Moderate sleep deprivation produces impairments in cognitive and motor performance equivalent to legally prescribed levels of alcohol intoxications' (2000), www.ncbi.nlm.nih.gov/pubmed/10984335/
30 M H Bonnet and D L Arand, 'We are chronically sleep deprived' (1995), www.ncbi.nlm.nih.gov/pubmed/8746400

easily irritated. And as if this isn't enough, our ability to handle stress decreases at the same time, at least until we pay off our sleep debt, which is not done just by sleeping for 8 hours the next day. It may take days to recover from, inhibiting us from using our stress management skills properly. In other words, we will feel more stressed and less able to handle it properly. This would reduce the efficiency of any strategy to handle our stress, so the first step is fixing our sleep.

Depression, anxiety and aggressive mood swings. A sleep-deprived brain tends to swing between positive and negative emotions. If the deprivation accumulates, those swings may even manifest as hallucinations or paranoia. Insomnia symptoms have been clearly associated with high levels of persecutory ideation, manifesting as anxiety, depression and paranoia.[31]

Don't take bad sleep habits as normal; they aren't. They would slowly but surely lead you to depression and anxiety.

Alterations of neurotransmitter receptors. Studies are indicating that, throughout the brain, neurotransmitter receptor expression and functions are sensitive to

---

31 Daniel Freeman, Katherine Pugh and Natasha Vorontsova, 'Insomnia and paranoia' (2009), www.ncbi.nlm.nih.gov/pmc/articles/PMC2697325/

sleep loss.[32] Some cases demonstrate that neurotransmitter receptors are affected rather dramatically by sleep deprivation.

We will cover this in more detail in the next book when genotype-specific stress management and how neurotransmitters dictate moods, motivation and overall wellbeing will be addressed. However, a quick explanation is that we *are* our neurotransmitters. They dictate our drive, motivation, learning ability and speed of thought, how organised our thoughts are and our moods. If our neurotransmitter profile is imbalanced or the corresponding receptors are altered, we will end up with a lack of drive, motivation, learning ability, processing speed etc.

How our health is affected by bad sleep

Beside its impact on our body and mind, bad sleep of course has an impact on our health. It can trigger or accelerate major diseases such as cancer or diabetes, impair our immune system and lead to all kinds of neurodegenerative diseases.

Cancer. Many studies have established a link between being exposed to light during nightshifts and higher

---

32 Fabio Longordo, Caroline Kopp and Anita Luethi, 'Consequences of sleep deprivation on neurotransmitter receptor expression and function' (2009), https://pdfs.semanticscholar.org/f0e7/10ae71ca169f1da667eac6609c347825f73c.pdf

cancer risks.[33] Cancer is the second leading cause of death worldwide and has been in a scary and continuous increase since the seventies. There are different reasons impacting on how prone we are to getting cancer, but bad sleep is surely a major one of them.

Diabetes. A study found that subjects who slept five or fewer hours were almost twice as likely to have incident diabetes over the follow-up period of ten years as those who slept 7 hours.[34] Diabetes is one of the major causes of death worldwide and is rapidly increasing. While the main causes of this type of diabetes seem to be related to nutrition and a lack of exercise, bad sleep increases the risk of becoming diabetic in the long term.

Accelerated aging. Living with a bad sleep habit is like driving down the highway of aging at full speed. The body will not have enough time to rebuild itself, which is the primary key to avoiding the majority of diseases. Low-quality or disrupted sleep results in the body releasing fewer rejuvenating hormones like melatonin and GH, which in turn accelerates the aging process.

---

33 S Davis and D K Mirick, 'Circadian disruption, shift work and the risk of cancer: a summary of the evidence and studies in Seattle', *Cancer Causes Control* **17**, 539–545 (2006), ttps://doi.org/10.1007/s10552-005-9010-9
34 James E Gangwisch et al., 'Sleep duration as a risk factor for diabetes incidence in a large US sample' (2007), www.ncbi.nlm.nih.gov/pmc/articles/PMC2276127/

Even our skin is not spared from the adversity of impaired sleep. A study indicated that chronic poor sleep quality is associated with an increase in the intrinsic signs of aging, such as diminished skin-barrier function and lower satisfaction with appearance.[35] Poor or insufficient sleep shortens the time period that the body is in self-repair and rejuvenation, accelerating the aging process.

Increased inflammation. A lot of studies with different set-ups and methods have shown the same results: sleep deprivation leads to a general increase in inflammatory markers such as cytokines and c-reactive proteins.[36] Chronic inflammation is the gateway to major troubles like diabetes and cardiovascular diseases.

Leaky blood-brain barrier and neurodegenerative diseases. An increase in inflammatory properties due to sleep loss can lead to an impairment of the blood-brain barrier (BBB) in the long run. The inflammatory markers attack the BBB which becomes leaky, leaving the brain prone to the risk of developing neurologic and neurodegenerative diseases.[37] Although research is promising that neurodegenerative diseases might be reversible, this research is in its infancy and there

---

35 P Oyetakin-White et al., 'Does poor sleep quality affect skin ageing?' (2014), www.ncbi.nlm.nih.gov/pubmed/25266053
36 Janet M Mullington et al., 'Sleep loss and inflammation' (2010), www.ncbi.nlm.nih.gov/pmc/articles/PMC3548567/
37 G Hurtado-Alvarado et al., 'Blood-brain barrier disruption induced by chronic sleep loss: low-grade inflammation may be the link' (2016), www.ncbi.nlm.nih.gov/pmc/articles/PMC5050358/

is still no medicine or treatment method. Prevention is key and sleep is a major part of prevention.

Impaired immune system. If you want to understand the link between your immune system and sleep, remember the last time you were sick. Because your immune system is busy fighting intruders, the first thing your body asks for is more sleep. Prolonged sleep deprivation and the accompanying stress response lead to a persistent production of pro-inflammatory cytokines and immunodeficiency.[38] Both have detrimental effects on health.

Obesity. Sleep is an important modulator of neuroendocrine function and glucose metabolism. Sleep loss has been shown to result in metabolic and endocrine alterations, including decreased glucose tolerance, decreased insulin sensitivity, increased evening concentrations of cortisol, increased levels of ghrelin, decreased levels of leptin[39] and hence increases hunger and appetite.[40] Every one of those alterations can result ultimately in obesity; the combination of all will just hasten it. Obese persons are at a high risk of all kinds of diseases.

---

38 Luciana Besedovsky, Tanja Lange and Jan Born, 'Sleep and immune function' (2011), www.ncbi.nlm.nih.gov/pmc/articles/PMC3256323/
39 Ghrelin and leptin are not two hobbits; they are the main hormones managing hunger and satiety. The first one, released by the stomach, is the hunger hormone and stimulates appetite; the second is released by fat cells and does the opposite.
40 Guglielmo Beccuti and Silvana Pannain, 'Sleep and obesity' (2011), www.ncbi.nlm.nih.gov/pmc/articles/PMC3632337/

Cardiovascular disease. In addition to being a major cause of high blood pressure, sleep deprivation shuts off the release of human growth hormone (HGH) which surges during sleep and is a great healer. This leads to an impairment of the inner lining of the blood vessels, which is the first step towards atherosclerosis and blood vessel ruptures.

Plaque building up due to calcium deposits is a further degradation in cardiovascular health due to sleep deprivation. Cardiovascular diseases are the number-one killer worldwide and sleep has a major impact on how prone we are to such diseases.

Infertility and decreased libido. Inadequate sleep decreases libido and increases the chance of both females and males becoming infertile. Sleep deregulation, circadian dysrhythmia, and activation of the hypothalamus, pituitary, adrenal (HPA) axis (a series of glands secreting hormones and belonging to the endocrinology system), all of which result from inadequate sleep, negatively alter fertility via pathways such as hormonal imbalances, reduced melatonin and increased inflammation.[41]

---

41 Jacqueline D Kloss et al., 'Sleep, sleep disturbance and infertility in women' (2014), www.ncbi.nlm.nih.gov/pmc/articles/PMC4402098/

ANNA'S CASE

A client of mine told me about his wife, Anna. He explained to me that Anna, a bright and straightforward person, had never experienced any anxiety attacks, paranoia or hallucinations until she was sleep deprived. Over a two-year period, she had experienced a difficult pregnancy followed by a baby who slept for no more than 90 minutes before waking up to be fed. After waking, Anna wasn't able to fall asleep again.

No one in Anna's family was aware of any bizarre behaviour until she had an aggressive anxiety attack which broke her down while preparing for a short holiday. She became concerned that she hadn't packed all necessary items into the cases and her husband would be angry with her. After that, her husband explained to me, she swung between being scared and crying and being happy and laughing many times.

We started right away with a supplementation protocol to reset her neurotransmitters. After just one night of good sleep, Anna was finding confidence in herself again. She had still needed to wake up many times during the night, but the protocol meant she was able to fall back into deep sleep right after feeding her baby. This made a big difference to her moods and wellbeing the day after. In parallel, and as a long-term strategy, we worked on reducing her stress input to the absolute minimum to help her recover and focus only on her baby.

3
What Good Sleep Can Do For You

'Sleep is the only sedentary activity, which protects from weight gain.'
— Chaput JP, Klingenberg L Sjödin[42]

Besides delaying the onset of diseases or acting as a power healer by reducing inflammation and supporting the body's repair mechanisms, good-quality sleep has far-reaching benefits. It has a major impact on our cognitive function by boosting neurogenesis, enhancing memory and balancing hormonal and neurotransmitter profiles. Good-quality sleep erases bad experiences on one hand and stores useful experiences for life on the other.

---

42 J-P Chaput; L Klingenberg and A Sjödin, 'Do all sedentary activities lead to weight gain: sleep does not' (2010), www.ncbi.nlm.nih.gov/pubmed/20823775

How our body recovers with good sleep

As much as sleep has a bad impact on our bodies when it's compromised, it works wonders for us when it's sound.

Athletic performance and risk of injuries. When a study on the impact of sleep on athletic performance implemented several interventions, including sleep extension and napping, sleep hygiene and post-exercise recovery strategies, it found that sleep extension had the most beneficial effects.[43] Adequate sleep also enhances motor-skill memories, which makes the athlete better in their sport day after day[44] and reduces their risk of getting injured doing the sport.[45]

Overall energy. I like to think of sleeping as filling a water tank and daily activities as draining water from that tank. If your sleep doesn't refill your tank enough, because it's too short, interrupted or of poor quality, you won't have enough to drain from it the next day and you'll have to push on your adrenals with coffee and stimulants to squeeze the last drops out of it. Ideally, your sleep restores more energy than

---

43 D. Bonnar et al., 'Sleep interventions designed to improve athletic performance and recovery' (2018), www.ncbi.nlm.nih.gov/pubmed/29352373
44 N Armstrong et al., 'International Olympic Committee consensus statement on youth athletic development', *British Journal of Sports Medicine* 49, no 13 (2015), 843–51.
45 M D. Milewski et al., 'Chronic lack of sleep is associated with increased sports injuries in adolescent athletes', *Journal of Paediatric Orthopaedics* 34, no 2 (2014), 129–33.

your day drains, so your day doesn't empty your tank completely, leaving some safety margin.

Heart health. A study by Harvard University on 23,000 people aged between twenty and eighty-three years has shown that 37% increased their risk of death from heart disease after quitting regular napping.[46] This effect was especially strong for the working population with a risk increase of more than 60%, so don't underestimate what even a short nap on a regular basis can do to help prevent the top killer, cardiovascular disease.

Coronary health. A study found a clear association between sleep duration and coronary artery calcification.[47] An hour's more sleep per night decreased the estimated odds of calcification by 33%.

How our mind recovers with good sleep

Good-quality sleep has an amazing impact on our mind. Besides being a natural healer of depression and psychiatric illnesses, it boosts our memory and decision making and increases our ability to manage stress.

---

46 A Naska et al., 'Siesta in healthy adults and coronary mortality in the general population' (2007), www.ncbi.nlm.nih.gov/pubmed/17296887
47 Christopher Ryan King et al., 'Short sleep duration and incident coronary artery calcification' (2009), www.ncbi.nlm.nih.gov/pmc/articles/PMC2661105

Neurogenesis. One of the most spectacular findings of modern research, pioneered by Dr. Michael Merzenich, is neurogenesis and brain plasticity.[48] Many people still think that we are born with a certain amount of neurons (nervous system cells) and nothing can alter this amount apart from age, which has an impact on increased cognitive decline, dementia and Alzheimer's disease. Of course, this is not true.

We produce new stem cells daily, which can develop into neurons and play a role in our cognitive function. This is called neurogenesis. There are certain activities which support neurogenesis and help produce more neurons, and there are others which reduce neurogenesis or stop it altogether. I'm sure you've guessed right – good-quality sleep helps regenerate our cognitive function as it ensures fresh neurons are produced and protected to grow. Sleep deprivation does the contrary.[49] Sleep also enhances insulin-like growth factor (IGF-1), brain-derived neurotrophic factor (BDNF) and GH, all of which are promoters of neurogenesis.

Neurotransmitter balance. Nothing drains neurotransmitters and creates imbalances more than an accumulation of inadequate sleep. When our neurotransmitters are imbalanced, we are imbalanced as well. The more imbalanced we are, the less we feel

---

48 Dr Michael Merzenich, *Soft-wired, How the New Science of Brain Plasticity Can Change Your Life* (Parnassus Publishing, 2013).
49 Carina Fernandes et al., 'Detrimental role of prolonged sleep deprivation on adult neurogenesis' (2015), www.ncbi.nlm.nih.gov/pmc/articles/PMC4396387/

like ourselves. Balanced neurotransmitters mean we are home, we feel splendid, our drive and motivation are through the roof, we are happy and see everything positively, even if it is stress.

Neuroprotection. Melatonin, which is known as the sleep hormone, has neuroprotective properties among its diverse functions. Different studies have shown that optimised melatonin levels help protect neurons by scavenging endogenous free radicals, activating several antioxidant enzymes and preventing programmed cell death.[50]

Delayed onset of Alzheimer's. A study has shown that when sleep disorders are successfully treated, cognitive decline can be significantly slowed down. The onset of Alzheimer's disease can then be delayed by five to ten years.[51]

Stress management and depression. Enough good-quality sleep achieves wonders in terms of stress management.[52] The brain, by intentionally erasing information related to stress and negative experiences, helps massively to reduce stress loads induced by bad experiences or trauma, so proper sleep hygiene

---

50 J C Mayo et al., 'Melatonin prevents apoptosis induced by 6-hydroxydopanine in neuronal cells: implications for Parkinson's disease' (1998), www.ncbi.nlm.nih.gov/pubmed/9551855
51 S Ancoli-Israel et al., 'Cognitive effects of treating obstructive sleep apnea in Alzheimer's disease' (2008), www.ncbi.nlm.nih.gov/pubmed/18795985
52 Andy R Eugene and Jolanta Masiak, 'The neuroprotective aspect of sleep' (2015), www.ncbi.nlm.nih.gov/pmc/articles/PMC4651462/

not only prolongs alertness and memory recall, it also relieves stress and depression.

Enhanced memory. During NREM sleep, our newly acquired information is copied into the long-term storage area of the brain, the cortex, where it may stay for the rest of our life. The hippocampus is then emptied and refreshed to acquire new information the next day.

This process is like copying the contents of a secure digital card (SD) into the computer's hard drive. A short sleep is the equivalent of pulling the SD card out of the reader before the copying process has finished. Short sleep after learning new information will ultimately lead to much of that information being lost.

By napping or having a long, good-quality sleep, we make sure newly acquired information is saved and our short-term memory is kept ready to receive new information.

Good-quality sleep, especially starting early evening, will also help with memory retrieval. Research has shown that people have a much better ability to remember things after a restoring and NREM-rich deep sleep.[53]

---

[53] S Ackermann and B Rasch, 'Differential effects on non-REM and REM sleep on memory consolidation?' (2014), www.ncbi.nlm.nih.gov/pubmed/24395522

Enhanced decision making. You probably don't feel this until your decisions impact something crucial. Jeff Bezos, Amazon's boss, says he makes sure to sleep 8 hours every night as not to risk making poor executive decisions the day after. He also keeps 'high IQ' meetings only in the mornings even if they would have to wait until the day after.[54] Regular 8 hours' sleep keeps your brain sharp as it has enough time to regenerate, rejuvenate and recharge.

Healing psychiatric illnesses. Patients suffering from depression, bipolar disorder, schizophrenia and other maladies may want to consider proper sleep hygiene as part of their healing strategy as the brain's glymphatic system clears out toxins and helps maintain cognitive function.[55]

How our health improves with good sleep

Good-quality sleep doesn't pass us by without healing us. It helps us detoxify, reduce chronic inflammation, repair our tissues and even cure major diseases such as cancer and diabetes.

Antioxidant. Good sleep reflects in healthy levels of melatonin, which is a powerful antioxidant. Deep, good-quality sleep of about 8 hours plays a big role

---

54 www.businessinsider.my/jeff-bezos-why-8-hours-sleep-important-when-making-important-decisions-2018-9
55 Andy R Eugene and Jolanta Masiak, 'The neuroprotective aspects of sleep' (2015), www.ncbi.nlm.nih.gov/pmc/articles/PMC4651462/

in fighting chronic inflammation and oxidative stress, both of which make us age faster and create the perfect environment for diseases, including cancer.

Anti-cancer. A good night's sleep may be one weapon in the fight against cancer, according to researchers at Stanford University Medical Center.[56] Their work is among the first to piece together the link between restorative sleep and recovery from cancer.

According to the researchers, the link acts in two ways: through melatonin and cortisol. Melatonin, the sleep hormone, has antioxidant properties and helps mop up damaging free radicals. Producing less melatonin due to poor sleep leaves the DNA more prone to cancer-causing mutations.

Cortisol, the stress hormone, helps regulate immune-system activity, including that of a group called natural killer cells that help the body battle cancer. In essence, people with disrupted circadian rhythms are more prone to cancer.

Anti-aging and tissue repair. During sleep, we secrete melatonin and GHs, both of which act as rejuvenation and anti-aging agents. Contrary to what bodybuilders may believe, injections of GHs are more effective at stimulating collagen formation in skeletal muscles

---

56 Stanford University Medical Center, 'Stanford research builds link between sleep, cancer progression' (2003), www.sciencedaily.com/releases/2003/10/031001060734.htm

and tendons than preventing muscle atrophy.[57] This suggests that a naturally occurring GH plays a big part in maintaining a collagen matrix, leading to the appearance of youthfulness.[58]

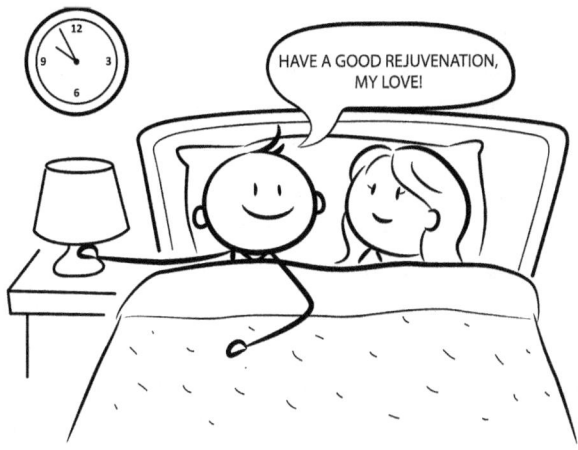

Insulin insensitivity. Since sleep, unless we're fasting, is probably the longest time period in our day that we go without food intake, the body has time to regulate blood glucose levels, regenerate insulin receptors and insulin secreting beta cells in the pancreas, and use fat for fuel. All of these enhance insulin sensitivity, which helps with glucose metabolism and keeps diseases such as metabolic syndrome or diabetes at bay.

---

57 S Doessing et al., 'Growth hormone stimulates the collagen synthesis in human tendon and skeletal muscle without affecting myofibrillar protein synthesis' (2010), www.ncbi.nlm.nih.gov/pubmed/19933753
58 The science of beauty sleep (2019), www.tuck.com/science-beauty-sleep

Hormonal imbalance. The master endocrine organ, the pituitary gland, which controls the secretion of hormones from the peripheral endocrine glands, is markedly influenced by sleep. First of all, during sleep, hypothalamic factors may be activated, as is the case for GH, or inhibited, as is the case for corticotropin-releasing factor (CRF). The other pathway by which sleep affects hormonal balance is via the modulation of autonomic nervous system activity. During deep sleep, sympathetic nervous system activity generally decreases and parasympathetic nervous system activity increases.[59] By having such an influence on the master endocrine organ and the autonomic nervous system, sleep plays a major role in our overall hormonal balance, including stress hormones by modulating the circadian rhythm, by GH release during the night time and by influencing the leptin and ghrelin secretion and thyroid hormones.

Detoxification. During NREM sleep, the so-called glymphatic system of the brain is working hard at disposing of toxic waste products and metabolites from the daily firing of neurons. A study has shown that brain cells reduce their size during sleep, allowing an increase of the intercellular space by up to 60%.[60] This allows for them to flush with cerebrospinal fluid to rinse toxic waste products, including β-Amyloid pro-

---

[59] Eve Van Cauter et al., 'The impact of sleep deprivation on hormones and metabolism' (2005), www.medscape.org/viewarticle/502825

[60] Dr Maiken Nedergaard, 'Neuroscience. Garbage truck of the brain' (2013), www.ncbi.nlm.nih.gov/pmc/articles/PMC3749839

tein, which is linked with Alzheimer's disease, out of the brain.

Better social appeal. And last but not least, proper sleep hygiene has been proven to make you look more attractive to others.[61] In a study, pictures of people were taken under exactly the same conditions – first after a period of good sleep, and then after a period of reduced sleep. The pictures were shown to a group of people who were unaware of the test circumstances. These people were less willing to socialise with a subject who was sleep-restricted. Sleep-restricted subjects were also rated as less attractive, less healthy and appearing sleepier compared to their well-rested selves.

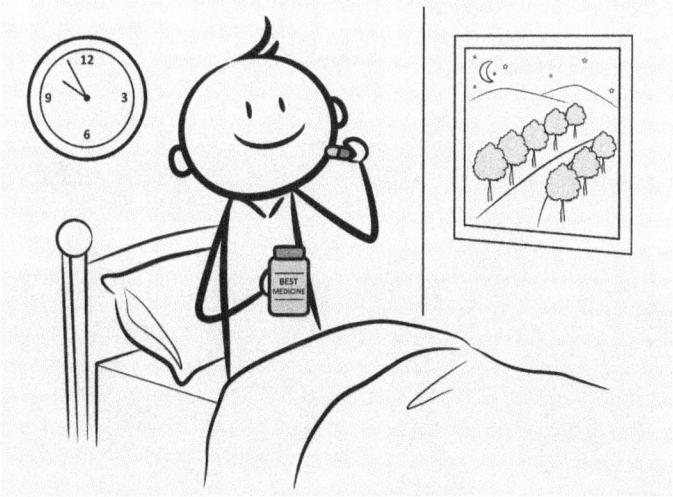

---

61 Tina Sundelin et al., 'Negative effects of restricted sleep on facial appearance and social appeal' (2017), www.ncbi.nlm.nih.gov/pmc/articles/PMC5451790

4
Techniques To Achieve Perfect Sleep In One Week – Quick Wins

'Your future depends on your dreams, so go to sleep.'
— Mesut Barazany

Now you are aware of the detrimental effects of bad-quality sleep and the marvellous benefits of rejuvenating sleep to your health and performance, let's learn some effective techniques to help restore your sleep in just one week.

Often people use smartphones and tablets to help them fall asleep. Others turn to medication or alcohol as a quick fix when they are overstressed and can't sleep. These are both false friends. They will not only disturb your sleep, they may also irreversibly damage your health.

For good-quality and uninterrupted sleep, prepare from the moment you wake up. In this chapter, I'll present some techniques I've adopted for my clients and myself. After only a few days of using them, we all achieved a balance in our sleep patterns and enjoyed having more energy during the day.

We're going to look at the four most important areas:

- Timing
- Nutrition and supplements
- Environment
- Mind and body

Timing

Timing is almost everything when you're trying to fix sleep. If you manage all other techniques properly but your timing is bad, then you will not fully benefit from your night's sleep even if its quality is good enough.

Here are a few techniques which will help you create the right time window for your good night's sleep.

Go to bed 15 minutes earlier each day. Do this each night until you hit your target. For example, if you normally go to sleep at around 11.30pm, it would take you eight days to hit a target of being in bed and going to sleep by 9.30pm. Once you've achieved your target, do everything in your power not to delay going to bed.

You may feel you have a valid excuse to stay up later sometimes, for example you have important work to finish. Work will never come to an end, but your health and performance will, so don't accept such excuses. Go to bed early as usual and reschedule unfinished activities for the next morning. Use your best window of time to complete important tasks, not your worst.

Anticipate. Always go to bed earlier than the time you wish to fall asleep. If you plan to be asleep by 10pm, which for me is the golden time, be in bed no later than 9.30pm.

Do you know what sleep has in common with a high-intensity training session? They may seem like opposites, but both need good preparation. Allow your system to shut down slowly. Dim the lights, read a relaxing book or just meditate. If you plan to be punctual, then you'll often be late.

Lower your activities towards the evening. Schedule your daily activities in accordance with your circadian profile. Your peak focus and concentration time is right after good-quality uninterrupted deep sleep. After this window, your focus will decrease throughout the day, with the worst time being the evening hours due to fatigue accumulation.

Prioritise the most concentration-demanding tasks in the morning. This prevents you from over-activating your brain prior to going to bed and inadvertently raising your cortisol levels at night.

Optimise your last meal. Macronutrients play a role in determining your sleep quality and quantity. Eating highly insulinogenic foods like starchy carbs impacts on blood-sugar and insulin levels, increasing your metabolism at a time when you wish to calm and rest your body. Sugary or highly spiced meals at the end of the day, along with alcohol consumption, tend to lead to fragmented sleep.[62]

We get similar results by consuming fructose. Even though it's not insulinogenic, which means it can't induce insulin release, fructose circulates in the blood until it's broken down into glycogen in the liver. If the liver is working a nightshift handling a fructose load, this might disturb your sleep quality or make you wake up in a sweat.

It's true that carbs in general help you release serotonin, which is the feel-good and relax neurotransmitter, so they help with falling asleep. But as my mentor Charles R Poliquin says, you need to deserve your carbs. A better mix for your last meal of the day would be fibrous vegetables, an easily digestible protein source like fish and smart fats to provide sustainable

---

62 *The Joe Rogan Experience* podcast, episode #1109 – Matthew Walker (2018).

energy and building blocks for the body during the night's sleep.

⏱ **Optimise your prime time.** The prime time for sleep preparation is the time between your last meal and the moment you fall asleep. Going to bed with a full stomach is not conducive to either the best quality of sleep or achieving your target on sleep hours. Your digestive system will be working a night-shift to produce all the acids and enzymes it needs to digest your food.

Conversely, going to bed too hungry won't work either. In this case, your instinct will be in survival mode, securing the building materials for your body rather than resting.

Find what works best for you. Your goal should be to fall asleep as quickly as possible and sleep without interruption until you hit your target of a minimum of 7.5 hours, or better still, 8 hours. As a rule of thumb, the prime time between eating your last meal of the day and going to bed should be somewhere between 2 and 3 hours. If you have a body composition goal, this may go up to 4 hours.

⏱ **Avoid napping in the afternoon.** As good as napping is, doing it at the wrong time can interfere with your good night's sleep or hinder you from getting to sleep on time. I advise you to schedule a nap before 4pm. If this time has passed, you need to avoid napping.

Keep the same sleep pattern throughout the week. Your body is conservative, preferring the status quo. It doesn't want to adapt to too many changes, which can hinder your peak performance.

One of the biggest dampeners on your performance is having a non-constant circadian rhythm. When you go to sleep later at the weekend, which is often the case for people who have a nine-to-five Monday-to-Friday job, you may find it difficult to return to your sleep routine during the week. Keep the same pattern at the weekend; don't disrupt your circadian rhythm!

Rise with the rooster. Don't wake up and be productive straight away, or worse, consume social media and news. The first thing you do in the morning will dictate your success during the day. Take some time early on to fuel your mind, meditate and plan. See every day as a new page in your life's book and prepare what you want to write on it. Use the first hour after you wake in the morning to focus on your coherence (see the technique 'Tune your heart in to coherence' in Part Two) and the main things you want to achieve today.

Waking up early is in sync with our circadian rhythm. Cortisol levels rise early to prepare to supply us with energy.

Nutrition and supplements

We are what we absorb. Of course, this impacts on our sleep quality, including how quickly we fall asleep and whether our sleep is interrupted or not.

Stimulant consumption and timing. Many people, depending on their culture, push themselves with coffee, tea or other stimulants to get ready for the day. A lot of Europeans like to drink coffee in the morning to get started and again after lunch when our digestive system is draining our energy, so we can feel sleepy. Then there is the 3pm coffee, which seems to help us finish the working day feeling wide awake. Some of us even consume an espresso right after dinner.

However, caffeine has a negating impact on our ability to nap or sleep soundly as it takes many hours to be flushed from the body. There are some who can drink an espresso just prior to going to bed as they are not caffeine-sensitive, but for the majority of the population, caffeine will impinge on our sleep cycle if we don't use it in harmony with the circadian cycle of our daily hormonal profile. Too much can also have a negative impact on our adrenals.

Depending on how your body responds to caffeine, limit your tea or coffee consumption to a maximum of two cups each morning. Avoid caffeine in the afternoon since your body needs up to six hours to neutralise its stimulating effects. If you are lucky and have the time to have a power nap, reduce your consumption to just one cup in the early morning and make it a special treat. I love to take my early morning espresso with a pinch of cinnamon, a pinch of stevia and coconut milk, or coconut oil if I want it black.

Reduce water consumption towards the evening. This is a good idea if you wish to avoid having your sleep interrupted by your full bladder. I like to reduce my water intake starting from 6pm, consuming only the water I need to take my supplements. If you find it difficult not to drink water immediately prior to bedtime, urinate before going to bed, even if you don't feel the need to. It's just a matter of damage limitation.

Alcohol won't help you. Avoid drinking alcohol in the evenings. Besides being a toxin, alcohol puts an additional load on the liver and may result in you waking up soaked in sweat – a result of overly high liver activity.

Alcohol may help you fall asleep quickly, but it interferes with REM sleep phases. Depending on the amount you have drunk, alcohol delays the onset of and the total length of REM sleep. It also reduces melatonin production.[63]

---

63 I O Ebrahim et al., 'Alcohol and sleep I: effects on normal sleep' (2013), www.ncbi.nlm.nih.gov/pubmed/23347102

Plan B when you wake too early. Have you ever woken up feeling ready for work, only to realise that it is only 4am? My preferred go-to supplement in this instance would be melatonin. The supplement I personally use is called Insomnitol. In addition to melatonin it includes 5-HTP, a precursor of serotonin, inositol, theanine and vitamin B6, which help to relax the nervous system and promote the natural ability to fall and stay asleep. If you take it, your sleep will be solid, but don't become too dependent on this supplement by taking it every night. I use it once in a while when I wake up too early or preventively when I know that I have a hard day ahead and I need to make sure I sleep well.

Magnesium. We are all deficient in minerals, especially magnesium and zinc. A good, absorbable type of magnesium, like threonate, or a mix of amino acids and magnesium chelates taken from mid-afternoon to just prior to bedtime will do wonders. This is my first technique if I want to instantly improve my quality of sleep without addictive side effects.

Magnesium is a mineral which we used to get mainly from natural mineral water. Today's water quality can't cover our needs, while at the same time, our needs have dramatically increased due to higher loads of toxicity, stress and carbohydrates consumption. Make magnesium supplementation a regular thing, not just a tool to improve your sleep.

Inositol. If a magnesium chelate such as threonate has helped, but isn't proving to be enough to get you to 8 hours of deep sleep, I would recommend you take inositol. Inositol is a B-like vitamin, which has potent anxiolytic and relaxing properties and helps with sleep. It will also help you set your neurotransmitters in balance.

Theanine. Theanine is an amino acid, which is extracted from tea and has calming or relaxing powers. When the effects of theanine were studied, the main result was that this rare amino acid induces an increase in the activity of alpha brainwaves.[64] Alpha brainwaves are extremely important to allow restoring relaxation. Without the so-called alpha bridge, we would be caught in the high frequency of beta brainwaves, which are more specific to chronic stress.

Environment

Our environment has a major impact on our sleep quality and deepness, how quickly we fall asleep and when we wake up. Here are a few techniques to help you create an ideal environment for the most rejuvenating sleep.

---

64 A C Nobre, A Rao and G N Owen, 'L-theanine, a natural constituent in tea, and its effect on mental state' (2008), www.ncbi.nlm.nih.gov/pubmed/18296328

Reduce electromagnetic field. An electromagnetic field (EMF) is generated by electrical devices or power cables. Nowadays, we live in a cloud of magnetism and wifi due to the power networks and connected devices we have all around us. I'm an advocate of having radiation-free zones, and what better place to start than in our own home?

Switch off wifi sources, smartphones, tablets and other electrical devices by shutting down the whole power supply at the electrical switchboard in your home. Except for the refrigerator and freezer, make sure all devices and wall power sockets are power free. Electrical radiation interferes in particular with deep sleep.

Displays will stress you. Exposure to light from display screens during the day but especially right before you sleep is a bad practice. Light in general can stress you out, but blue light does more so than other kinds. It hinders your brain from naturally producing melatonin, the sleep and rejuvenation hormone, while inducing cortisol production, the stress hormone. You end up tired and wired, which is not a good recipe for quality sleep.

The temperature effect. Sleep research has shown that bedroom temperature affects how quickly we fall asleep, and how long and well we sleep by decreasing the REM sleep.[65] The body, as a preparation mechanism for sleep, lowers its temperature, so a cooler room temperature will help you fall asleep more quickly and guard against sleep fragmentation. I won't give temperature recommendations as different people have different suitable temperatures, so you need to find out your ideal for yourself, but a couple of ways to speed up the time it takes you to fall asleep could be going to bed only in underwear or not covering yourself up to speed up the cooling process.

The light effect. Exposure to sunlight causes a natural process whereby the body attunes itself to start secreting melatonin after sunset. Exposure to blue light during the day and any light after sunset confuses your circadian rhythm, stopping the secretion of the sleep hormone and restarting the release of cortisol instead. Just avoiding artificial light will have a huge impact on your sleep quality and resultant energy levels during the day.

The solution here is to use blue-light-blocking glasses, which you can get from your optician, and dim all lights after sunset.

Sleep in a room as dark, cool and quiet as a cave. A cave is a perfect place for sleep. It has optimal humidity, cool temperature, no light and no sound.

---

65 Kazue Okamoto-Mizuno and Koh Mizuno, 'Effects of thermal environment on sleep and circadian rhythm' (2012), www.ncbi.nlm.nih.gov/pmc/articles/PMC3427038/

Establishing those conditions in your bedroom will help you improve your sleep quality and length massively.

Eliminating light from your bedroom is the first technique to try because it's highly effective. It works from day one and it's easy to implement. Not only can our eyes see light, our skin might be able to sense it too,[66] so if you want to eliminate sleep interruptions, this is a big step in the right direction. Shop around for blackout material, which is dunked in paint and 100% sealed, and it's inexpensive. Make sure you test it with a flashlight prior to cutting.

If you can't influence the noise coming into your bedroom, then your only option is to plug your ears. If you like something efficient and durable, you may wish to try Sleeep® or Sleeep® Pro.[67] I live right now in a windy region next to the sea and I use mine regularly when the wind is too noisy; I keep them under my pillow for easy access when they're needed.

Mind and body

As much as sleep has an impact on our bodies and minds, the converse is also true. Our sleep posture, hormonal and neurotransmitter profile and state of

---

66 N Hoang et al., 'Human and Drosophila cryptochromes are light activated by Flavin photoreduction in living cells' (2008), www.ncbi.nlm.nih.gov/pubmed/18597555
67 www.flareaudio.com

mind have an impact on our quality of sleep, how quickly we fall asleep and how deep our sleep can be.

Sleep posture. New research has shown that sleeping position has an impact on our quality of sleep. People sleeping on their left side tend to have nightmares, which can interrupt or disturb their sleep. This is believed to be due to the body trying to release the pressure other organs are putting on the heart. Sleeping in a supine position could lead to the jaw falling open, which forces mouth breathing, something we should avoid for different reasons, the main one being a decrease of CO_2 in the lungs which would lead to an impaired cellular absorption of O_2 due to the Bohr effect. [68].

Further research has shown that body posture has an effect on the efficiency of the glymphatic transport.[69] The glymphatic system is responsible for flushing toxins out of the brain while we're in deep sleep. The best posture to facilitate brain detoxification is the lateral position, so the lateral right side is the winner.

Take care of your serotonin levels. One neurotransmitter which plays a major role in relaxing us, inducing good feelings and sleep quality, is serotonin.

---

68 Patrick McKeown, *The Oxygen Advantage: The simple, scientifically proven breathing technique that will revolutionise your health and fitness* (Piatkus, 2015).
69 Hedok Lee et al., 'The effect of body posture on brain glymphatic transport' (2015), www.ncbi.nlm.nih.gov/pmc/articles/PMC4524974/

Serotonin is the predecessor of the sleep and rejuvenation hormone, melatonin. When serotonin is low, melatonin peak is low and sleep quality declines. Stress lowers the feel-good neurotransmitter serotonin, leading to bad sleep quality along with food cravings, depression and other mood disorders.[70]

As 95% of serotonin is produced by gut bacteria, taking care of your gut health will ultimately boost your serotonin levels and allow for high-quality sleep. Once your gut flora is reestablished, choose raw materials for the production of serotonin. Zinc, vitamin B6 and tryptophan, which is found in proteins like turkey, are key to maintaining healthy serotonin levels. As a supplement, 5-HTP, which is a precursor of serotonin, helps replenish healthy serotonin levels.

In Part Two, we will discuss in more detail how to establish and maintain a healthy gut flora.

Medication is for the sick. If your sleep is bad and you're thinking about resorting to medication as a first step, think again. Clinging to medication in the hope of solving your sleep issue is like shooting a mosquito with heavy artillery. You may fix the problem, but you'll be digging a deeper hole with each dose. No medication is devoid of side effects and regular ingestion can lead to addiction, which won't happen

---

70 Dr M Hyman, *Broken Brain Series*, Episode 5: Depression & Anxiety, www.brokenbrain.com

with natural supplementation such as magnesium or theanine.

Research has provided enough evidence regarding the harmful side effects of sleep medication. Besides causing cancer, increasing the risk of accidents, epilepsy and anxiety, it can kill you. The number of Americans killed every year by medication like zolpidem, temazepam, eszopiclone, zaleplon, triazolam, flurazepam, quazepam and barbiturates is almost as high as the number of people killed by smoking, 500,000 vs 560,000.[71] And even if you survive these nasty medications, they will make sure that your memory eraser is working optimally.[72]

Meditate and pray. If you have a religion, then practise your religion. Every religion has its own form of meditation, so don't fall into routines and rush through prayers. Use techniques for concentration and deep connection with yourself, such as correct breathing to achieve heart coherence (see the technique 'Tune your heart in to coherence' in Part Two). Feel the strength of your prayers and meditation connecting you with your Creator and the universe. Going to your source offers relief, fills you with joy and will culminate in

---

71 Daniel F Kripke, 'Hypnotic drug risks of mortality, infection, depression, and cancer: but lack of benefit' (2018), www.ncbi.nlm.nih.gov/pmc/articles/PMC4890308/
72 Hsin-I Shih et al., 'An increased risk of reversible dementia may occur after zolpidem derivative use in the elderly population' (2015), www.ncbi.nlm.nih.gov/pmc/articles/PMC4603066/

TECHNIQUES TO ACHIEVE PERFECT SLEEP IN ONE WEEK

helping you sleep in peace and having successful days.

If you don't follow a religion, then you can learn how to meditate. Using the proper breathing technique while meditating, as described under 'Tune your heart in to coherence' (Part Two), will massively help you to establish a state of heart coherence, to reduce stress levels and prepare for the day or the night sleep.

Earn your recovery. Being active in the right way will make you tired and help you sleep better at night. But of course, there are wrong ways to be active. If you go for a demanding workout late in the evening or take part in long sessions of aerobic training, your cortisol levels can be negatively altered. They may then peak when you are nearing your sleeping time.

Spread the word. Make an announcement and inform anyone who may contact you late in the evening that you go early to bed these days. Publicise it! This will ensure that they won't bother you during your sleeping time and help you commit to your goal of going to bed early.

Declare one hour prior to going to bed a time of absolute radio silence. Never reply to messages during this time. You need to let your circle of friends and family know that you are dead serious about your recovery time.

SPECIAL CASE: JETLAG

A time-zone change has a massive impact on your circadian rhythm. If you rely on it to return to normal by itself, it may take two weeks or more. Your body needs time to get acquainted with and acclimatise to the new time zone and can only do this at a slow pace. During long flights, your body gets dehydrated, and that doesn't help with the recovery process either.

Here are my strategies to bridge the gap:

- If the time difference is wide, start shifting your activities a few days before departure so your body can anticipate the change.
- Go training a few hours before flying. This makes you pleasantly tired and ready for napping during the flight.
- Make sure you are well hydrated prior to and during the flight. Don't rely on the airline staff to supply you with water; prepare an empty bottle with amino acids and electrolyte complex and fill it with water after the safety checks.
- Apply the technique of abstinence described in the chapter 'Managing Environmental Stress' in Part Two. Plug your ears and try to sleep or listen to a podcast. Using the illuminated screen will only stress you more and keep you wired.
- If you want to sleep because you will arrive at your destination early in the morning, take melatonin to facilitate in shifting your circadian rhythm.
- Upon arrival, get earthed. Walk barefoot or sleep on a conductive grounded mat to synchronise your body with the new location. This will help you

TECHNIQUES TO ACHIEVE PERFECT SLEEP IN ONE WEEK

quickly readjust your circadian rhythm in alignment with that of the new time zone.

- Schedule a training session for when you arrive. Go for a dense one-hour workout where you touch every muscle group combined with high volume work. The target is to get exhausted and remain pleasantly tired for the rest of the day.
- One hour prior to bedtime, my go-to supplement would be Insomnitol™ to reset my biological clock.

Although your body generally needs two or more weeks to adapt to the new time zone, these strategies will help you reset in one or two days.

Part One: Conclusion
Perfect Sustainable Sleep

'The general that sleeps the most wins the war.'
— Charles R Poliquin

If all the effects of rejuvenating sleep could be condensed into a supplement capsule, it would only be accessible to a few people because of its astronomical price. While we will probably have to wait a long time for such a supplement to become available on the market, sleep is free, accessible to everyone and entirely dependent on our own decisions and the priorities we set during the day.

I hope that you are now ready to take the right steps towards progressively restoring the quality of your sleep. Your benchmark should always be deep, good-quality sleep for 8 hours within your golden window.

For sure, you'll have distractions and priorities, but your inner controller should always bring you back to your benchmark. If your inner controller doesn't work properly, your distracted state becomes your norm.

If you achieve 8 hours of good-quality, deep sleep, you will set yourself up to fix 70% of health and performance problems. In Part Two we will dive into stress management, which will help you address the remaining 30%. But before we move on, let's take a look at just how effective sleep can be at battling disease.

AZAM'S CASE

Despite Azam's young age of fifty-five, he suffered from severe Parkinson's disease. His symptoms had started small and just on one side, then progressed with time until he was completely disabled, unable to speak or stand.

A few months after his surgery to insert a deep brain stimulator (DBS), I started managing his nutrition with the goal of helping him with his poor digestion. But my ultimate goal was to investigate how I could use nutrition or lifestyle changes to help him mitigate the effects of his disease.

During the interview, I quickly discovered that besides nutrition, sleep and stress management were the weakest links for him. Because his disease had made it difficult for him to socialise, he had started isolating himself and spending all his time on his mobile phone, watching videos until the early morning hours. His sleep was not only brief, as his kids would wake him up early, it was also interrupted. Azam was waking up many times to use the bathroom as he liked to drink tea long into the evening. In addition, he hated sleeping in darkness and would always have a light on.

Once we'd implemented a progressive restriction in mobile phone display use, I convinced him to switch off the light and limit his beverages in the evening, in combination with taking a high-quality magnesium supplement. He soon began sleeping for longer and his sleep was much less interrupted. The dietary changes and key techniques we then applied to handle his daily stress load helped return his circadian rhythm to normal, which is key to long and rejuvenating sleep during the night. He felt more energetic during the day, and best of all, showed significantly fewer symptoms of Parkinson's disease.

PART TWO
TWO WEEKS TO MASTER STRESS

Life needs the right amplitude and frequency of stress to be worth living, no stress or too much of it would both bring it to a dead end.

5
How Does Stress Affect Your Health?

Stop running after life, slow down and let life sprint after you.

Now we've addressed the wonder supplement of sleep, let's go into the details of stress management. But before we do that, it's worth mentioning one more time that there is no strategy to improving health and increasing performance, whether physical or mental, that doesn't have sleep as its main pillar. Without enough good-quality deep sleep, any strategy will ultimately fail. When your sleep is right, stress management becomes an easy game, so don't focus on stress management if your sleep is compromised.

In Part Two, we will define what stress is, introduce a few basics and some terminology, and discuss the

HPA axis briefly. This is the main hormonal mechanism behind the stress response. The stress response is an absolutely normal reaction from our body which regularly helps us achieve the hardest of goals and may even save our lives, but we will also look at when our stress response starts to become a burden on us.

Once we have done all this, we will discuss the emitter/receptor approach. This defines six major stress sources and provides actionable techniques to specifically reduce each stressor (getting the emitter side under control) while increasing our stress tolerance by strengthening the receptor side.

Stress keeps you alive

There are situations where a high level of stress can save your life. Staying cool in front of a hungry predator, for example, may not be the most appropriate thing to do if you are not contemplating suicide. You would need a quick surge of energy and clear cognitive function to cope with the situation and decide whether to fight or run for your life. Well, let's face it, it's more likely to be the latter.

The fight-or-flight mechanism was first identified by Walter Cannon,[73] but situations in which we would need to use it are rare now as we are not living the

---

73   T M Brown and E Fee, 'Walter Bradford Cannon' (2002), www.ncbi.nlm.nih.gov/pmc/articles/PMC1447286/

same life as our ancestors. We don't have the same need to protect ourselves from life-threatening situations, but we have much more stress than our ancestors ever had. We have created this stress ourselves with our advanced lifestyle. Our ancestors' sources of stress could be counted on the fingers of one hand – predators, rival tribes, weather and, if they were really unlucky, lightning or earthquake.

There is a side of stress which makes us more robust for life, and this is not a bad thing, so our strategy to manage stress needs to help us minimise unnecessary stress, but it's not about eradicating stress altogether. That's an impossibility anyway.

Stress is similar to internal friction inside a car engine. That friction generates heat which the engine needs to meet its full range of power and performance, but too much internal friction would dramatically decrease its performance and may lead to malfunction.

How stress works

Imagine trying to manage stress levels with a swinging pendulum. The pendulum is made of a steel ball and a length of rope, and it needs a certain level of stress to keep swinging. Without this stress, the pendulum will stand still.

Any external stress which is not in sync with the pendulum will temporarily disturb its oscillation, but eventually the stress will increase the oscillation after stabilisation. Think about recovering from the emotional pain of a divorce or the physical pain of an injury. But should this stress be too much, the pendulum might reach an irreversible state, eg it could break or fall over, which would be the death of the oscillation.

Before we dive into stress management with its multiple aspects, let's have a look at some stress-related terminology.

Genotype. This is your genetic makeup. It influences your body's physiology and, more specifically, your central nervous system (CNS), so it affects your character and temperament.

Stress. Every input, either external or internal, triggers a cascade of stress responses from the brain. On the physiological level, every input triggers the HPA axis with neurotransmitter and hormonal release by the adrenals.

Stressor. This is the stress emitter or source of stress. It can be anything from a hungry lion to an unpleasant sound, a toxin in your blood stream, your bank account status, artificial light, your child misbehaving, a bad meal, your boss having a meltdown, your beloved sports team losing etc.

Stress load. This is the amplitude of the stress input. It includes:

- A base load if the stress is the input we deal with regularly
- A stress ramp if the stress load is higher and longer lasting than the base load
- A peak stress if the stress load is short in time and maximum in amplitude

Stress tolerance is our ability to absorb stress without triggering a stress response. When we, for example, accumulate stressful loads without solving anything and closing the episodes, or if our neurotransmitter balance is not well-established due to poor nutrition or sleep habits, we inadvertently lower our tolerance to handling stress. In these cases, a stress input with low amplitude can trigger a massive avalanche of a reaction.

The stress response. This is how we react to a particular stress input. It depends on our actual stress load, genetics and neurotransmitter balance. Whatever the source of stress, the physiological process that the body uses to respond to it is the same. The adrenals release the catecholamines adrenaline and noradrenaline and the cortisol hormone with the ultimate goal of ensuring survival. This process can be our friend when we require short bursts of energy, but it can also be our long-term enemy if we misuse it and rely on it too much to push us through an overly stressful life.

It is normal to have a higher concentration of cortisol in the morning hours. This is a natural body function to provide us with enough energy to kick start the day. It's also normal during a workout to provide our muscles with enough energy to go through the demanding programme, and it's essential to survive a fight-or-flight situation. But it's not normal to have too high a cortisol level in the afternoon or late evening or to have chronically elevated cortisol levels. Chronic stress is the fastest way to age.

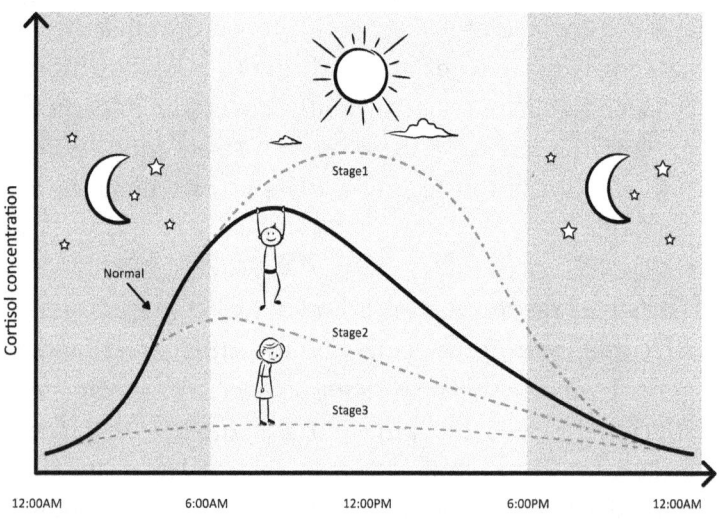

The curves in the illustration show increasingly unhealthy circadian profiles. In the healthy circadian rhythm, the cortisol level is at its lowest between midnight and 3am. It starts to increase from there and peaks around 8am. An abnormal circadian rhythm starts with an increase in cortisol secretion during the day, as shown by the curve relating to stage 1. In stage 2, the adrenals start to reduce cortisol release, which is the body's attempt to put on the brakes. Finally, in stage 3, only a flat, low distribution of cortisol remains throughout the day.

It's worth mentioning here that melatonin has its peak around 3am, when cortisol is at its lowest, and falls continuously to reach the daytime levels when cortisol is at its peak around 8am.

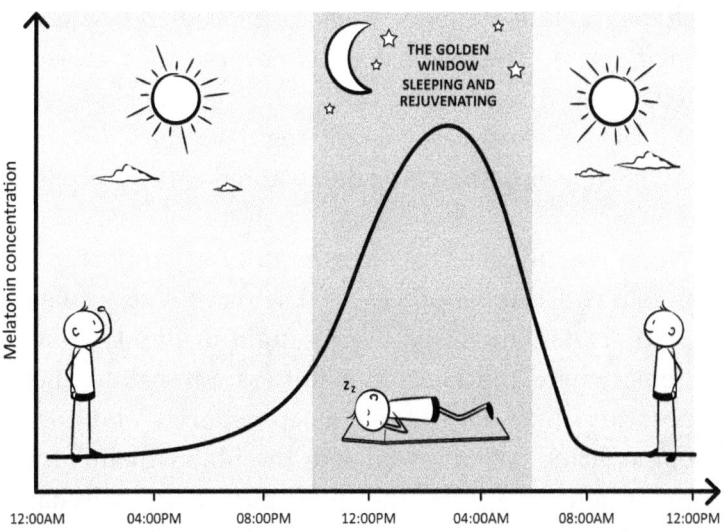

HPA axis

To better understand the physiological process behind cortisol response, we need to have a look into the HPA axis in more detail. Let's come back to our hungry predator. When we see a fierce predator approaching, our brain receives a picture from our eyes and starts the stress cascade by sending a signal to the hypothalamus gland, which sits within the centre of the brain. The hypothalamus then releases the corticotropin-releasing factor (CRF). This is received by the pituitary gland which sits just below the hypothalamus. The pituitary gland then releases the adrenocorticotrophic hormone (ACTH) which is sent to the adrenals to trigger the release of cortisol. The adrenals are pyramid-shaped glands sitting on top of the kidneys, hence their name. The whole cascade works in a closed loop control manner, which means the brain senses the released cortisol levels and regulates the CRF and ACTH release to fine tune the required cortisol levels.

When we have instant stress input, our body reacts in two consecutive processes. The first process takes place instantaneously during fight-or-flight situations, where the neurotransmitters adrenaline and noradrenaline, also known as epinephrine and norepinephrine, are released into the bloodstreams by the adrenal medulla (the inner part of the adrenal glands). It leads to raised heartrate, constriction of blood vessels and an increase in blood pressure. The second process, which takes a few minutes to occur, involves the release of the cortisol hormone by the adrenal glands cortex (the outer part of the adrenal glands).

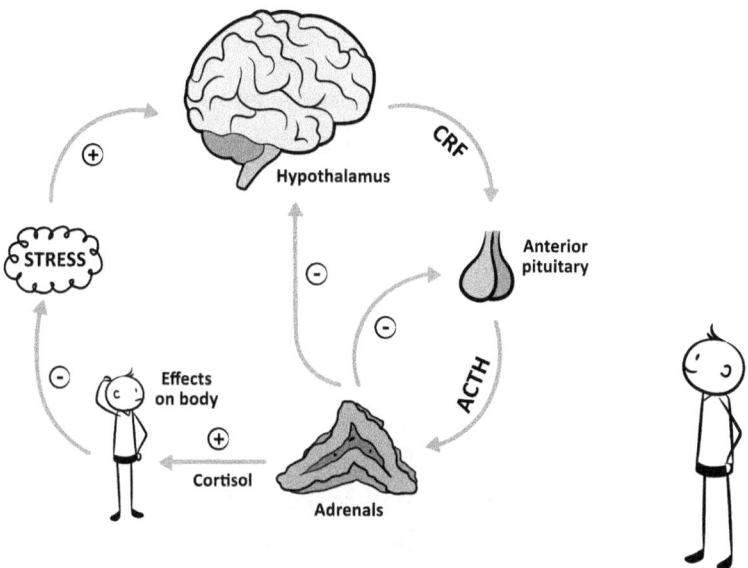

The cortisol dilemma

The good side of cortisol and the catecholamines, adrenaline and noradrenaline, is the release of energy when we require it. In a fight-or-flight situation, cortisol and catecholamines will guarantee the release of the required energy, even if they do this by temporarily shutting down the immune system and inflammation. Our brain doesn't care about the immune system as it needs to ensure our survival.

In a fight-or-flight situation, cortisol and catecholamines will:

- Release glucose into the bloodstream
- Supply glucose to the brain by temporarily increasing the body's insulin resistance
- Increase the heartrate to supply enough nutrients to all body parts and vital organs
- Dilate pupils
- Slow down digestion
- Suppress the immune system
- Relax the bladder

During a long period of cortisol release, as in the case of fasting, the cortisol will make sure that there is a continuous supply of glucose into the bloodstream.

Of course, there is a bad side to cortisol. Prolonged exposure to stress will increase the concentration of cortisol in the body throughout the day (see stage 1 in the earlier illustration). This chronically high cortisol level will break down muscle tissues and inhibit muscle synthesis to produce the much needed amino acids.[74] Furthermore elevated cortisol levels will kill

---

74 P S Simmons et al., 'Increased proteolysis. An effect of increases in plasma cortisol within the physiologic range' (1984), www.ncbi.nlm.nih.gov/pmc/articles/PMC425032

brain cells, shrink the brain and lead to dementia.[75] Unbalanced ratio of cortisol to dehydroepiandrosterone (DHEA) hormones also reduces our androgen levels, including testosterone.

If exposure to stress is long lasting, or if we tend to amplify our stress responses and live in a stress cloud, the adrenal glands will sooner or later slow down cortisol production (see stages 2 and 3 in the curve). This situation is known as adrenal insufficiency.

The term adrenal fatigue is also used to describe this stage of lowered cortisol production, but this is not correct. Adrenals don't fatigue, they just lower their production because of upstream physiological processes. The correct medical term is adrenal insufficiency or Addison's disease.[76]

Other results of adrenal insufficiency are chronic fatigue and fat storage in the lower abdomen. But as my mentor and friend Christian Maurice correctly describes it, it's not the adrenals that should be blamed, but the stress we put upon them, either psychologically or physically.

Because cortisol increases glucose levels in the blood to ensure energy supply, chronic stress means chronically

---

[75] Dr M Hyman, *Broken Brain Series*, Episode 2: Gut Brain Connection: Getting to the root of a broken brain, www.brokenbrain.com

[76] Todd B Nippoldt, 'Is there such a thing as adrenal fatigue?' (2017), www.mayoclinic.org/diseases-conditions/addisons-disease/expert-answers/adrenal-fatigue/faq-20057906

high glucose levels. The body will counteract this by releasing more and more insulin to bring glucose levels to normal. Then we have two endocrine axes acting against each other, resulting in hyperglycaemia and insulin resistance and putting us at a high risk of becoming diabetic. Research has also shown that an exposure to chronically elevated cortisol levels will have a negative effect on different parts of the brain by causing neuronal shrinkage and inhibiting neurogenesis.[77] Moreover, a high cortisol level depletes the neurotransmitter serotonin by increasing its uptake, creating a neurotransmitter imbalance.[78] Serotonin is important for our brain's balance and good moods.

Chronic cortisol levels slow down the immune and digestive systems. Besides accelerating aging and promoting inflammation in the whole body, stress increases our risks of health problems like sleep disorders, hypertension, cardiovascular disease, weak immune system, autoimmune disease and insulin resistance.

---

77 Bruce S McEwen, Carla Nasca and Jason D Gray, 'Stress effects on neuronal structure: hippocampus, amygdala and prefrontal cortex' (2016), www.ncbi.nlm.nih.gov/pmc/articles/PMC4677120/
78 G E Tafet et al., 'Correlation between cortisol level and serotonin uptake in patients with chronic stress and depression' (2001), www.ncbi.nlm.nih.gov/pubmed/12467090

6
The Sources Of Stress

'It's not the load that breaks you down, it's the way you carry it.'
— Lou Holtz

Generally our stress response is so complex, we have to break it down into different aspects with specific approaches to better understand it in the first place, and then come up with the best practical solutions. There are two fundamental approaches to managing stress, the emitter/receptor approach and the genotyping approach. Both approaches are interlinked to give us a different view on the mechanisms of the same stress process and offer different actions to bring our general stress management skills to the next level. In this book, we will be concentrating on the emitter/receptor approach.

In terms of the possible stress sources, let's differentiate between genetic stress, lifestyle stress, social stress, financial stress, environmental stress and nutritional stress. As always in life, there is no definitive black and white answer, so these sources of stress may be interlinked in some way.

Let's identify each one of these sources in more detail.

Genetic stress

You're likely to know in your circle of family and friends if some people are more prone to stress. They tend to overreact with their stress responses and can even be a source of stress for the people dealing with them by being super anxious and making mountains out of molehills all the time. Others tend to take it easy by playing down the same stressful situations or ignoring stressful input altogether.

Think about this kind of stress as sunlight reflecting on a surface. If the surface is a concave mirror, it will intensify the sun's light and induce combustion. If it is flat, it will just reflect the light without being a big influence. But imagine a surface which is convex, like a mirrored ball. It will diminish the light density and play it down so much that we can look directly into the powerful sunlight on this surface without harming our retinas.

But I caution you here not to treat your genetics as a 'get out of jail' card. We are our genetics, but our genetics are not us. We can influence them by making the right choices and responsible decisions in life. Our genes can be activated, stay dormant or even corrected depending on the behavioural choices we make day to day in life and in our routine.

Lifestyle stress

This is stress which is induced by our lifestyle choices. It might be how much time we spend looking at the TV, PC, smartphone etc. If every five minutes, we're looking at our mailbox or timeline on our mobile phone, it's obvious we will gradually increase this stressful load over the day.

This kind of stress is self-induced. It results from the bad situations we have put ourselves in and impatience or unrealistic expectations from ourselves and others.

Social stress

This is the type of stress which results from our interactions with other people in our surroundings. Those people might be our children, partner, neighbours or colleagues. This kind of stress might run along a steady plateau, like dealing with our kids misbehaving or partners arguing, or it might peak, like when being fired or we lose a loved one.

Financial stress

Most of us have some sort of financial stress, regardless of our social status. We strive to have more, and at the same time fear losing what we already have.

Usually people who live without being able to save or accumulate vast wealth know how to deal with finances because they have to ensure their daily survival. They have a continuous stressful load to cover their day-to-day needs. The more we have, the more likely we are to be anxious about losing it, the less we'll trust our environment and the more isolated and lonely we'll become as a result. We may fear for our kids when they go to school; we may trust people less and think everyone who is kind to us has ulterior motives; we may fear that our business will be adversely affected when we are on holiday or busy elsewhere. Show me someone struggling to make ends meet who cares about hedge funds, fluctuating gold and oil prices. They likely won't have sleepless nights should the market drop.

I'm not saying people without a load of money have less stress; they may be struggling to keep a roof over their heads or feed their kids. What I want to highlight here is that we can't solve all of our financial stress; whatever our financial status, we will probably just switch our load to another kind of financial stress.

Environmental stress

This type of stress is brought on by our environment. Just as we feel relaxed when we look upon a scene of natural beauty or listen to the sound of waves on a beach, we can be stressed by a concrete jungle with police sirens screaming and car horns blaring endlessly.

This source includes every kind of stress that comes from the environment we are in and can sense. There might be toxins in the air which overload our body, noise or artificial light which stress us, and EMF or radioactivity damaging our cells. EMF is one of the biggest contributors of stress today.

Nutritional stress

There are three distinguishable kinds of stress related to nutrition. The first one is nutrition quality – whether what we consume triggers inflammation and allergies. The second is our response to the consumption of stimulants like caffeine or alcohol, and the third kind is due to prolonged fasting.

We will address each of these stress sources further later in the book, but for now you can go to www.phpstrengthclinic.com/stress and take the Peak Performance Stress Test to see where you are on the scale. Find out what your particular stress sources are and what to focus on first for peak performance and recovery.

The emitter/receptor approach

In a nutshell, within a stress process, there are always two sides: the emitter and the receptor. The emitter is where stress is generated – our environment, social scene, lifestyle, nutrition etc. The receptor is how we receive stress, process and respond to it. This depends mainly on our genetics, neurotransmitter make up and habits, which influence and, to a certain degree, define us.

In the emitter/receptor approach, the ideal strategy for dealing with stressful loads is to aim to work on both sides of the equation. On one side, we should work on our environment and all its identifiable stress sources, and on the other side, we work on ourselves. Managing the emitter side and getting it under control, we put ourselves in a better situation with the least stressful input. Strengthening the receptor side makes us more robust and resilient when dealing with stress loads.

Think about these two aspects as a castle. A wooden castle built on soft sand would survive in a friendly environment, but the same castle would quickly be overrun in a hostile environment. What we want is an indestructible castle in the friendliest of environments.

The genotyping approach

This approach looks into the different personality types with the aim of helping us discover our own nature and those of our counterparts. Knowing our genotype and our partners', family members', friends' and colleagues' genotypes will give us an edge over them when we're dealing with stressful situations. It is a tool which will allow us to control the way we process stress, for example, by increasing our stress tolerance, and then enable us to successfully deal with others and minimise their stress input on us. The genotyping approach makes use of established personal assessment models to define the different genotypes.

Now we have identified the most common sources of stress, let's dive into each source and the techniques for managing them with respect to the emitter/receptor approach. Focus on one technique at a time. The techniques are presented from quick wins to sustainable long-term results. Start with one which will be the easiest for you to implement and let it become a part of your routine and lifestyle. Once it's fully integrated, move on to the next easiest. Prioritise the ones which work quickly and bring you the speediest results to rapidly improve your capabilities at handling and managing stress. This will increase your stress tolerance and make you more resilient while putting you in a better position to focus on the next techniques with long-term success.

7
Mastering Genetic Stress – Immediate Wins

'The greatest weapon against stress is our ability to choose one thought over another.'
— William James

Don't use your genetics as a convenient excuse to justify not doing anything about your stress response. It's all in your hands, so to speak. You can follow your genetics and react as you wish, but you can also learn and apply some easy but effective steps to help you better control how you receive, process and respond to stress.

The decisions we make while processing stress are crucial as they form the way in which our genes express themselves. This will define which genes will be activated, which ones stay dormant and even which ones will be corrected. Yes, you read that right. As in many areas of epigenetics, we are able to correct our genes if we successfully bring our behaviour under control and apply some effort towards making the right choices.[79]

As you are reading this book, the chances are high that you have already started making those choices. Let's look now at how to break genetic stress down, starting with those all-important immediate wins.

Ignore it

If we ask ourselves whether we really need to respond to every stress input that we sense, we will soon recognise that there are some stresses we have no need to eliminate to achieve peak performance. Still, way too many people fall into the trap of worrying non-stop about all eventualities their brains can imagine, and the more creative they are, the more they find to worry about. People who tend to do this keep themselves busy all the time doing nothing, and as a result, they get more used to stress and their sensory function recognising new stress inputs becomes more efficient with time.

We have to teach ourselves, step by step, to increase our stress tolerance by ignoring unnecessary stress

---

79 Barry M Lester et al., 'Behavioral epigenetics' (2011), www.ncbi.nlm.nih.gov/pmc/articles/PMC3783959/

inputs and sensing when there is no value in triggering our stress processing mechanism. In other words, we need to sharpen our senses to be selective towards which stress inputs are worth exploring and replying to, while ignoring and filtering out everything else.

Here is an effective technique to apply. Prior to processing any stress load, ask you yourself the 3-second question:

Is there any added value to me replying to this stress load?

If your answer is not a resounding yes after 3 seconds, move on. Save your cortisol levels, time and mood for a more serious case.

You will require patience to ignore some stress inputs and move on, but by applying this filter, you may eliminate a large portion of your stress load anyway. Don't allow parasitic stress loads to trigger your stress response; raise the bar and only respond to the cases that deserve your attention.

Change your position or activity

If you are hyper-stressed, change your position or location. If you are lying on a bed, sit down, and if you are sitting, then stand up and walk about. Changing the position you were in when you felt stressed helps you break from that stressful situation and change your thought processes quickly. Often, going out for a walk in the fresh air improves your mood and helps you make better decisions.

Meditation, proper sleep and deep, slow breathing techniques will all help with this kind of stress too.

Fake it until you make it

If we are afraid or scared, we make ourselves small and activate our flexor muscle groups like chest, abdominals, biceps, hamstrings etc. The converse applies – when we feel good, motivated or happy, we tend to make ourselves big and tall by opening our chest and spreading our arms. We may even jump in the air. In this case, we activate our extensor muscle groups such as our back, neck, triceps and quads. Our hormonal and neurotransmitter profiles have an impact on how our body behaves. That's nothing new; it's an instinct we're born with.

> 'Rise and rise again until lambs become lions.'
> — *Robin Hood* (Ridley Scott movie, 2010)

What is new is the effect of our body and posture on our hormonal and neurotransmitter profiles, and as a result our stress levels, moods and wellbeing. The way we stand, move and hold our arms and torso impacts on our self-esteem, testosterone and cortisol levels.

This is what Dr Amy Cuddy discovered from her research a few years ago.[80] Just standing and raising our arms in a V while we're in a stressed or inconvenient situation in which we would normally make ourselves small will raise our testosterone by 20% and decrease our cortisol levels by 25%. Try this easy technique for yourself – it works for many of my clients.

Sense when you need time

We as humans like fast action and accomplishment once we've focused on something. The same applies to solving our problems or when we're dealing with stress, but sometimes it's better to allow time to play its role and let things settle down. Rushing to solve every issue we encounter may over-complicate things or induce more stress. Take patience as gold and rushing as silver; sense when you need to take a step back and wait, freeze all thoughts and leave time to play its role.

There are of course times when you need to fix things right away. In these cases, giving them time won't do any good. Train yourself to evaluate each stress input and act accordingly. Use your discretion.

---

80 D R Carney, A J Cuddy and A J Yap, 'Power posing: brief nonverbal displays affect neuroendocrine levels and risk tolerance' (2010), www.ncbi.nlm.nih.gov/pubmed/20855902

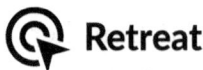 Retreat

Taking yourself off on a retreat alone once in a while will open your eyes and help you get out of the forest to see the trees. A retreat could be a two- or three-day holiday surrounded by nature, or take a look through a telescope or microscope to wonder at creation.

Solitude can and does rejuvenate. It will put you in a position to re-evaluate your life, including your relationships, job and current situation. This short and controlled separation will prompt you to see the real value of what you have and help you stop taking all of the bounties life has to offer for granted.

Tune your heart in to coherence

When we think about intelligence, we tend to think about the brain as the centre of human intelligence, but that's actually not quite true. We have neurons in our intestinal tracts and in our hearts too.

Our heart, with its 40,000 neurons, has its own cognitive function and is at the centre of human intuition and smart intelligence. It has its own nervous system with long- and short-term memory and even neurogenesis. But what really makes our heart so special is its ability to emit the strongest magnetic field in the body, which can be measured from a few metres away.

The various research works of Dr Lew Childre and his team have shown that when we're experiencing negative emotions such as anger, frustration or anxiety, our heart rhythms become more erratic and disorderly.[81] In contrast, positive emotions, such as appreciation, love or compassion, are associated with highly ordered or coherent patterns in the heart rhythms. As part of the research, Dr Rollin McCraty describes heart coherence as a state of increased harmony and stability in higher level control systems in the brain; increased synchronisation between heart and brain, and in the activity occurring in the two branches of the autonomic nervous system; and a general shift in autonomic balance towards increased parasympathetic activity, also known as vagal tone.

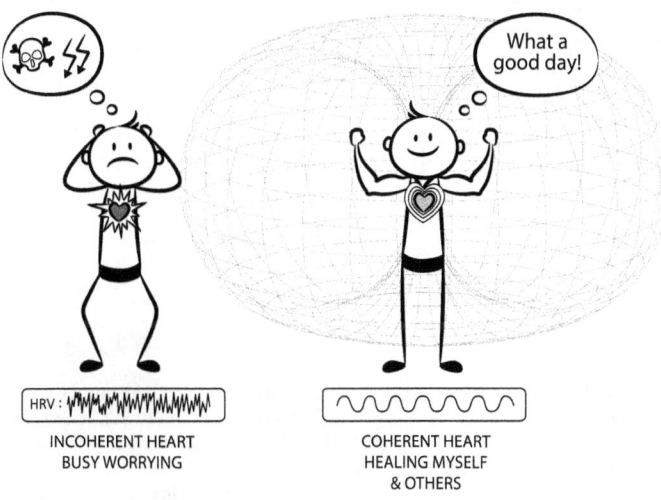

---

81 L Childre et al., *Heart Intelligence, Connecting with the Intuitive Guidance of the Heart* (Waterfront Digital Press, 2016)

When we are in a non-coherent state, there is no balance between our heart and our brain, or between our sympathetic and parasympathetic nervous systems. We then tend to have a louder inner noise and make bad decisions, which produce even more stress.

Another finding of the research is that a person's brainwaves show a degree of synchronicity with EMFs produced by another person's heart through hand touching, as in handshakes, and amazingly without touch.[82] But the latter is only true when the receiver's heartrate is in a coherent state. This means people, like other animals, are able to intuitively sense another person's heart state and synchronise with them.

A third finding has shown that EMFs generated by the heart may have direct effects on DNA conformation and cellular growth when the heartrate is coherent with an intention to produce the given change,[83] which is extremely interesting. The most amazing thing is that this enhances healthy cell growth by 20%, while inhibiting the growth of tumour cells by 20%.

---

[82] R McCraty, 'The energetic heart: bioelectromagnetic interpretations within and between people' (2003), www.researchgate.net/publication/274451622_The_Energetic_Heart_Biolectromagnetic_Interactions_Within_and_Between_People

[83] G Rein and R McCraty, 'Local and non-local effects of coherent heart frequencies on conformational changes of DNA' (2001), www.semanticscholar.org/paper/LOCAL-AND-NON-LOCAL-EFFECTS-OF-COHERENT-HEART-ON-OF-Mccraty/a0d9fca1c5cda01fcd2897fc-c8a31f2836346af7

'There are as many healers in this world as human beings.'
— Dr. Randoll[84]

All these findings clearly indicate that humans and animals are connected via our magnetic fields prior to using our five senses. With positive feelings – love and compassion – we can harmonise our heart's state to coherence, which is transmitted outside our bodies to positively influence other people. The second key finding is that those same magnetic fields are able to produce biological effects and heal both us and people around us.

Now to the question of how to tune your heart in to coherence. Well, that's easy: proper breathing and positive thinking. The same lab that conducted the research I've just shared also came up with a tried-and-tested breathing technique called The Quick Coherence® technique,[85] which allows us to achieve a coherent state in about one minute. Alternatively, you can check out my power breathing technique.

Power breathing

One of the first things we learn in our mother's womb is breathing. In a similar way to our heart beating,

---

84 Dr U Randoll, www.youtube.com/watch?v=Ypigj0oCfMM (www.dr-randoll-institut.de)
85 www.heartmath.org/resources/heartmath-tools/quick-coherence-technique-for-adults

breathing is one of the most intuitive habits we have. We don't have to think about it to do it continuously, even if we are asleep.

Unfortunately, as intuitive as it is, breathing is also one of the most neglected performance enhancers. Proper breathing is crucial to physical and mental performance due to the enhanced oxygen uptake, which helps massively as a stress management tool.

Let's have a look at some facts about breathing:

- The heartbeat decreases when we exhale because of the parasympathetic nervous system being activated.
- During the inhaling phase, the sympathetic nervous system is activated and our heartbeat increases.
- Fast, shallow breathing, known as hyperventilation, leads to insufficient oxygen enrichment of the red blood cells (RBCs).
- Hyperventilation leads to the loss of too much carbon dioxide, too. Carbon dioxide is crucial for the release of oxygen from the RBCs, so the RBCs will have a hard time releasing oxygen to the cells where energy is produced.
- Mouth breathing produces less pressure loss compared to nose breathing so leads to the loss of too much carbon dioxide and dehydration.

- Nasal breathing ensures the right air humidification, heating and filtering of small particles, and helps increase our tolerance to carbon dioxide. Increased tolerance to carbon dioxide will in the long run allow us to decrease our breathing frequency and amplitude, which has a direct impact on us achieving maximum oxygen consumption (higher VO2 max) during aerobic efforts and higher levels of calmness and reduced stress when at rest.

- Nasal breathing also supplies the lungs with nitric oxide (NO), which is produced in the nasal cavity and plays a major role in dilating air tubes and blood vessels.

We can come up with a protocol which allows us to lower stress levels while increasing our oxygen uptake, tolerance for handling carbon dioxide and overall performance, including maximum oxygen consumption. In general, we have to inhale deeply for a relatively short time to minimise the activation of the sympathetic nervous system, and then take longer to exhale to activate the parasympathetic nervous system instead. This will allow us to swiftly reduce our heartbeat and the stress response. Then we need to increase our time with a high level of carbon dioxide to increase our tolerance to it. Avoiding breathing through the mouth will help us keep our carbon dioxide high, which helps with oxygen uptake.

It's better to use this technique while lying on your back with one leg extended and the other at flexed at about 90 degrees. In this position, you will be more likely to relax the maximum amount of muscles. Close your eyes and breathe deeply through your nose using your diaphragm to lift your chest and lungs. Take a short time to inhale a maximum amount of air into your lungs. Hold the breath for few seconds prior to exhaling, then take as much time as possible to exhale. Progress with each breath by pausing for longer before inhalation and taking longer during the exhalation phase. Push the boundaries with each breath until you absolutely have to move on.

You can of course use this technique while seated if it's inconvenient to lie down. Be sure to sit comfortably. Drop your shoulders and then pull them backwards, and keep your spine straight.

If it's inconvenient to sit, then breathing deeply while standing is also possible. In this case, I would suggest keeping the spine straight by raising the chest, bringing the shoulders back and dropping them, and keeping the hips in a neutral and comfortable position. Raise your arms up to the sides while inhaling. Your arms should be at about 45 degrees to your sides with palms up when you reach maximum air content in your lungs. Hold them there before you breathe out post inhalation, then turn your hands palm downwards and exhale slowly while bringing your arms down. Your arm movements and breathing should be synchronised.

I would recommend you apply this breathing technique many times during the day to reduce overall cortisol levels and relax, and especially immediately after peak stress input. In the case of an acute peak in stress, such as a fight-or-flight situation, don't wait. Start this breathing technique right after the stress input to supply the body with more oxygen, bring the heartrate to a normal pace and make sure you're highly stressed for as short a time as possible.

These are the wins you can incorporate into your life straight away to start managing your stress. Now let's move on to the wins that will keep you going for the long term.

8
Mastering Genetic Stress – Long-term Wins

'If you treat every situation as a life and death matter, you'll die a lot of times.'
— Dean Smith

Now we have looked in detail at the techniques you can use to master your stress immediately, let's delve into some long-term wins to keep you going for the rest of your life.

Remain childlike

I often ask myself what we should do to avoid taking everything too seriously. After all, when a situation has passed, often we realise it wasn't worth the stress.

Children are best at not taking everything so seriously. They have a totally different perspective towards stressful input to adults, mainly because their stress input is much lower than ours. I'm not implying that they don't have any stress load at all, as they do, but they are able to filter a lot out and process what remains much more efficiently than us.

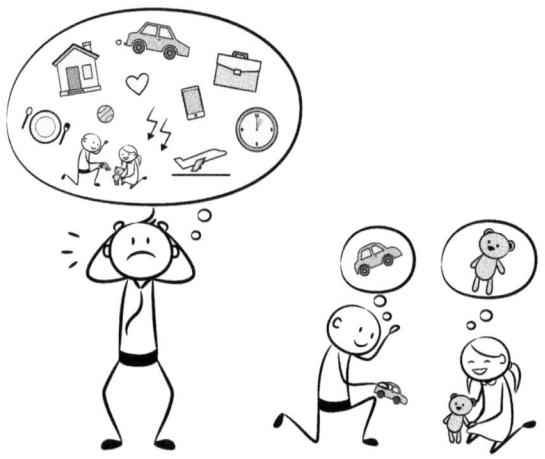

What can we learn from children?

1. They treat everything as a game.

2. They are masters at living in the present and are noticeably less focused on the future than adults. They don't really care about the past at all as they have forgotten most of it anyway.

3. They have innate innocence.

4. They are not good multi-taskers, which allows them to have only one worry at a time. Even if they are possessive and materialistic, they recover in record time once they get their ice-cream. Adults tend to whine and moan for far longer and about different things at the same time.

5. They are motivated and excited to explore new things and take on new challenges. While they are excited and happy, they are too busy to take stress inputs seriously.

6. Their reset button after a good sleep works much more efficiently than ours and they start a new page every day. We adults tend to carry our worries over from day to day.

A mix of strengths and weaknesses make children masters at stress management. They receive less stress load than adults because of their reduced attention or perception, and if they do receive stress inputs, they recover quickly once they get what they want.

It's up to you to choose what you wish to accept. For my part, I know that I will always be a kid deep within.

Learn optimism

What's going to hit you will hit you, no matter how protectively and well you act, and it will likely make you stronger. What's destined to miss you will miss you, even if you do everything wrong.

A study on 999 subjects over 10 years has shown that being optimistic about life could halve the mortality rate compared to being pessimistic.[86] Another study reviewed different types of evidence and their impact on longevity, with the main results showing that life satisfaction, optimism, positive emotions and absence of negative emotions lead to better health and longevity.[87]

Ask yourself if you're a stress inducer

There are people who seem to have a never-ending ability to produce enough stress for their entire social circle. This extreme situation is a result of an accumulative process that has been going on for years where individuals neglect their health, sleep, nutrition and exercise, which leads to imbalanced neurotransmitter and hormonal profiles. This tends to mean they never review or rethink their behaviour. When this becomes a routine, it can have an impact on their character. They receive so much stress without positive processing, they become the stressor themselves.

---

[86] E J Giltay et al., 'Dispositional optimism and all-cause and cardiovascular mortality in a prospective cohort of elderly Dutch men and women' (2004), www.ncbi.nlm.nih.gov/pubmed/15520360

[87] Ed Diener and Micaela Chan, 'Happy people live longer: subjective well-being contributes to health and longevity' (2011), https://doi.org/10.1111/j.1758-0854.2010.01045.x

It's like a vessel of water getting heat input all the time. One day, the connected safety valve will blow. As long as the vessel doesn't receive any care, its safety valve will continue blowing, depending on the heat input.

This stands as a warning to us against neglecting our brain balance, which mainly depends on sleep, nutrition and exercise, and not to use our genetic makeup as a passport to do as we like. It's our own choice to continue with or to break out from this routine. We can attend to any aspects of life which we have neglected for too long. We can fix our sleep and nutrition and re-establish our brain chemistry. In the worst-case scenarios, we may need to consult a competent psychologist, but it can still be done.

Before you get that far, though, ask yourself whether you are a source of stress. Then ask loved ones whether they are a source of stress on themselves. We don't change ourselves overnight, except in the most dramatic of cases. Rather, change is so slow, we sometimes don't even feel it, so make a point of asking this question every few months. This will help to ensure you don't change in negative ways.

Never complain

Complaining has never solved any problems. On the contrary, it tends to prolong the stress input by making us, along with those we are complaining to, more angry, agitated or anxious. Nobody likes to be with people who complain because in the long run it can isolate us, particularly from positive people who could elevate us. They detest the negativity which emanates from people who spend most of their time complaining.

If we make something bad into a habit, we risk facing big troubles when we want to change it later on. The more we complain, the more efficient our neurons will be at firing together to follow the brain map responsible for complaining, and the harder it becomes to get rid of it. We will feel an urge to complain that will become stronger with time, even if we have no reason for complaining.

Instead of complaining, regard the issue as a challenge and just have one thing in mind: how to solve it. Once it's solved, learn from the experience and make sure you don't encounter the same situation the next time around.

Be grateful and forgive

We humans as a species are excellent at adapting to new situations and circumstances in life. We establish our routines quickly to feel good and secure. This is our survival instinct, but too often our routines overrule everything in life, including the situations we should be grateful for rather than taking for granted.

We take our health, wealth, education, freedom and peace for granted, forgetting how fortunate we are and that others have worked hard or even sacrificed their lives for us to be in the position we are in today. Often, rather than being grateful, we complain that we have far less than others.

My trick here is easy, but massively powerful. Stop for a second, take some time out from your life's hassles and think. Think about adverse situations others are in and be grateful for the rest of the day.

Let me give you few precise examples. They are intended to help you break your routine and sharpen your sights to see all that is good in life.

- Imagine the happiness a couple in their forties would feel if they had been trying for a baby for many years and are looking for the first time at the ultrasound pictures of the foetus. Many people take having kids for granted.

- Imagine a family stopping their kids' education because they can't afford to send them to school anymore. Many people take their kids' education for guaranteed.

- Imagine a family has had to flee a war and leave everything behind. Too many people take peace and freedom for granted.

- Imagine a family going hungry night after night. Often, the food people throw away could feed that starving family for days.

Count your blessings and be grateful for what you have and where you are. This is something we can do without any physical or financial effort, and it can have one of the biggest impacts on our moods. Just saying thank you in a sincere way raises our dopamine levels and makes us instantly happy, but it does take training to become efficient at being grateful and make it a habit.

Look out for any opportunities to say thank you sincerely. There are always plenty of opportunities to be grateful to yourself and, if you believe, to God. You can start by thanking yourself for putting in the hard work and being resilient and patient over the years you've spent studying or working. Be grateful for the nice weather, for your health, and for material and non-material things. Be single-minded about this and practise it regularly as it will elevate you and boost your dopamine levels to make you a person who others like to spend time with.

Hand in hand with being grateful is being able to forgive. This is not a sign of weakness, as some may think. On the contrary, it's all about true strength of character. Forgive, but don't fall into the trap of being confronted by the same situation again.

Fight the right fight

If you were a king, which option would you take? Would you choose to fight every soldier in every army to conquer the world, or would you focus on the kings of other places and take everything and everybody in one single fight?

I'm talking about fighting, yes, but not in the way you may think. What, then, do I mean by this primitive analogy? Let's define the roles here.

The king is your inner-self and the whole army represents all the enemies you may encounter in your life. Don't bother fighting every single one of them; focus on one fight with the king. If you win over your inner self, then you will win over all others, but if you waste your energy fighting everyone else, you will become a slave to your inner self and to them too.

Sweet past, unknown present, scary future

We generally have a much better relationship with our past than our present and, even more so, our future. The past is under control and unchangeable. Nothing can happen to it anymore. We often keep good memories from the past; even if we remember hard times, we see them as a jolt which made us stronger. But we tend to feel unsure about now and what tomorrow might bring.

Imagine you are in a garden. There's a well behind you and the sun is shining above you. You need the right amount of water to keep your plants alive, so your labour and the sun will make them grow. But you don't want to use an excessive amount of water, otherwise you'll flood your garden, and you certainly don't want to climb down the well to live in the dark and the damp. On the other hand, you can't stand the full sun for too long while working in your garden.

Your well represents your past, your garden represents your present and the sun represents your future. The moral of the story is to use your past as a well of experience and have your future in sight, but live your now. The past is what made you who you are, and you need to have a plan for where you want to be in future, but focus on the present and own it.

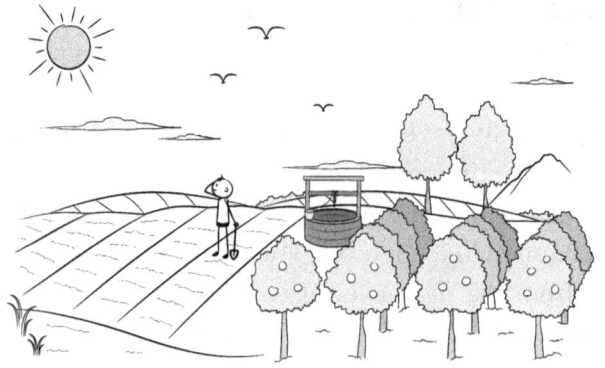

By the way, exposing the retina indirectly to the morning sun has huge positive impacts on physiological processes in the body, but that's a story for another book.

Change your perspective

When you're problem-solving, assume your point of view is wrong and change your perspective by looking at the problem from a totally different angle. Take some time to do this efficiently and distance yourself from your original perspective. Often, the only perspective we use in solving problems is our original one, which essentially means it is narrow.

> 'No problem can be solved from the same level of consciousness that created it.'
> — Albert Einstein

There are no problems, just challenges

Our attitude dictates the direction our problem-solving takes. If we say, 'Oh, problem', our stress response mechanism kicks in and lasts until we've found the antidote or solution. If we see challenges, our stress response mechanism still kicks in, but this time our dopamine and testosterone levels rise too to take on that challenge and overcome it.

Never focus on the problem, but rather on the targeted outcome. Don't tell yourself lies, believing you're no good at something or you can't do it; take the challenge. There is no failing, just learning.

Similar to a heavy squat, where our eyes are looking is where the trajectory of the lift will go, as our eyes dictate the direction. If we're looking to the ground our cheek will end up squeezed between the bar with the 1RM load and the spot we have been fixating on. Open your chest, look up over the horizon, breath in, squeeze every muscle you have, feel your strength, and challenges will be sweet.

Master doing nothing

This is not easy for someone who is into and all about peak performance. Doesn't the peak performer have to be on the go all the time? No, actually, the peak performer needs time windows of doing nothing productive. The idea behind this is to effectively change their mind and push the reset button.

I once asked my mentor Charles R Poliquin – the most successful strength and performance coach on earth[88] – for his best methods to manage stress. His answer was surprisingly simple. He regularly dedicates some

---

88 Measured by the count of Olympic medals and world records in 28 different sports he coached, and his impact on the strength and performance world.

time to an activity that is all about fun. It has to be a non-productive activity, otherwise it will miss the point. Ideally it will be an activity that doesn't use any electronics.

The best activities are those you do outside and/or with your kids/friends/family. You need to do your chosen activity/-ies regularly enough to balance out your stress load, so relying on your yearly holiday is a bad plan as it is too infrequent. Ideally, take part in your activity daily for a short period of time or weekly for a slightly longer period of time to be effective.

Don't overthink things

There are people who tend to overthink simple things and make them complicated. Usually, solutions are easier than we think they are; it is just that we overthink them. Simplicity and clear thinking are the keys to solving any issue.

Nothing worthwhile grows within our comfort zone. To grow, we need to be ready to do things others fear to do. This separates the men and women from the children, so to speak. Don't overthink it when you're faced with hardships; step forward and confront the fear.

> 'In the middle of difficulty lies opportunity.'
> — Albert Einstein

Use your imagination

Recent research, especially from neuroscientist Dr Michael Merzenich,[89] who is a pioneer in the field of brain plasticity, shows that our brain is not rigid. This means neurons are not linked to a certain function or body part for life; they can change and adapt depending on how they are used.

One of the core ideas of neuroplasticity is that neurons that fire together wire together in one map. The more often a person has the same thought, makes the same decision or follows the same actions, the better the neurons responsible for this particular action will be at firing together and the more efficient the person becomes at it. In the context of managing stress, the more often we have negative thoughts, make average decisions or perform undesirable actions, the harder it gets to deviate from them. On the other hand, if we regularly have positive and wholesome thoughts, even if they are imaginary, the better we will get at being positive, less stressed and more well balanced.

This is extremely important. Positive thoughts are powerful and effective tools to remodel our mindset and help us overcome difficult and stressful situations by remapping our brains. Psychiatrist Jeffrey Schwartz makes use of the plasticity of the brain to successfully treat his patients in the case of obsessive compulsive

---

[89] Michael M Merzenich et al., 'Brain plasticity-based therapeutics' (2014), www.ncbi.nlm.nih.gov/pmc/articles/PMC4072971/

disorder (OCD), for example, which involves extreme worrying without obvious reasons.[90]

The basic idea is to first recognise that the deceptive negative thoughts are not part of you, because you are not that kind of person. As soon as those deceptive thoughts emerge, focus on something positive such as a success story or enjoyable experience, even if the deceptive thoughts are still present. By doing this, you force the brain into rewiring itself to a new brain map, which ultimately links to the initial situation. With sufficient training, the brain gets so efficient at this that the positive thoughts take the upper hand rather than the deceptive thoughts. This method can be used to overcome anxiety, depression, anger or addiction.

JOSEPH'S CASE

Joseph is a university professor and a father of three. His wife describes him as a bright man, well balanced in life and highly respected by his colleagues and family members. Joseph has never had any close friends or hobbies as he has always been dedicated to his work and family. He has also never exercised or done any labour-intensive work before. For a period of over thirty-five years, he was either at the university busy teaching his students, or at home busy teaching his kids.

When his wife hired me to help, he was still respected by his colleagues and loved by his students, but he had

---

90 R Gladding and J M Schwartz, *You Are Not Your Brain: The 4-step solution for changing bad habits, ending unhealthy thinking, and taking control of your life* (Avery, 2012).

developed a serious case of chronic anxiety. This made him a real source of stress for his wife and children, and absolutely unsupportable. Worrying had become his first hobby and second profession. He would see absolutely everything in a negative light and was set against anything new. For him, the best-case scenario would be all his family members safe home with the door locked and no one even thinking about going into the dangerous outside. He worried about eventualities, and was very creative at that.

Interestingly, not one of his colleagues or students noticed anything was wrong except for the fact his hair had turned white. He was efficient at playing the same role he had done for decades and hiding his anxiety. Such a huge shift in personality had taken a long time to develop, and the incremental changes were so small that no one had seen anything coming, and therein lay the danger. When we don't stop from time-to-time to do a self-review, our genetic expression can shift from balanced to over-worried and we can become a huge source of stress for ourselves and our family.

As if this was not enough, Joseph had developed a serious case of OCD and would wake up a number of times during the night to check that the gas valve was still closed. This worsened his stress levels since he couldn't recover during the night.

Joseph's case needed time and a long-term strategy. He needed to look into all possible aspects of the complex situation, but without scaring himself. When he came to me, we could only start by implementing tiny changes in nutrition/supplementation and lifestyle to enhance his sleep, reduce inflammation, strengthen his immune system and establish better hormonal and neurotransmitter profiles. This helped him reduce his anxiety and regain his smile and motivation.

After a while, he became more happy and positive about life and less scared when his kids went to school or were away over the weekends etc. Joseph is now, after five years of continuous follow up, much more balanced and happy. He has even started telling his famous jokes again, which is a good indication that his mental health and satisfaction are where they should be.

As extreme as Joseph's case may seem, people are too often falling into routine traps and adopting habits which accumulate slowly over time and may ultimately end with them experiencing similar conditions.

Your routine is your descendants' heritage

There was some interesting research done on a group of mice and their descendants.[91] Some mice were shown a cherry every day, and right after that they were given a gentle electric shock. After this group of mice gave birth, the researchers repeated the experiment and showed their offspring a cherry. Guess what their reaction was? The young mice reacted in exactly

---

91 B G Dias and K J Ressler, 'Parental olfactory experience influences behavior and neural structure in subsequent generations' (2013), www.ncbi.nlm.nih.gov/pubmed/24292232

the same way their parents did. They were scared and released a load of cortisol.

This test was carried out on many generations descended from the initial group of mice and the behaviour was found to have been passed down from one generation to the next. And the same applies to humans too.[92]

The moral of the story is that we need to be careful about the decisions we make and the things we do and allow to become our habits. We become our habits, our genes become our habits, and this is not just limited to us. We can pass bad habits through our genetics to our descendants.

You have been warned!

---

[92] Irene Lacal and Rossella Ventura, 'Epigenetic inheritance: concepts, mechanisms and perspectives' (2018), www.ncbi.nlm.nih.gov/pmc/articles/PMC6172332/

9
Mastering Lifestyle Stress – Immediate Wins

'There is more to life than increasing its speed.'
— Mahatma Gandhi

This type of stress is brought on by our lifestyle choices, including the use of electronic displays, the way we organise ourselves and prioritise our work, the kind of sports we do and how we perform them, and how we handle our expectations. We may inadvertently be putting ourselves under a stress load that is entirely self-inflicted.

In this chapter, we will discuss some techniques we can implement to mitigate our self-inflicted stress straight away.

First activity dictates your day

The first task you do in the morning will dictate your whole day. If you start by grabbing your phone to check email and timelines, you are likely to continue doing this for the whole day. Don't allow negative social media and bad news to contaminate your day's creativity. All your focus in the first hour of your morning should be on two things: your heart, especially your coherence (see 'Tune your heart in to coherence' in Chapter 7), and the new day ahead. Start your day on the right foot – meditate, read a book, schedule your time – to ensure you finish strongly.

 Learn effective organisation

If you are disorganised, you are contributing vastly to your own stress load and adding to the loads on others in your daily life and environment. The good thing is it's never too late to learn to be organised. Put things where they belong, be minimalistic and separate yourself from things you don't need. Schedule your time ahead, finish tasks prior to moving on and perform your job to your best ability. Don't procrastinate and ignore outstanding tasks. Those are just a few approaches and strategies to start working on in your organisation.

Being organised means you're always prepared for any eventuality, whether it is a new task, a new challenge or an unexpected event. As you have done your homework and are prepared, you will free your mind to focus on and deal with a new stress load. Your life, working and living environment, relationships etc won't add to it. Rather, they will support you to perform better and master the stress you are under.

If you don't have this support, you'll have disorganisation. You possibly won't realise it because you are creating it and living within it, but without any buffer against stressful loads, your temper will be short and you will overload quickly in difficult circumstances. Being organised in your working and living environment increases your tolerance for handling stress and will give you more of a crumple zone to mitigate it.

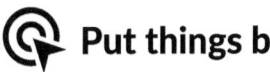 Put things back

If you can remember the second law of thermodynamics, you will understand one crucial thing: entropy, which quantifies our level of organisation, will decrease with time, except if we put work in. In other words, if we put no work into a system, our disorganisation automatically increases.

If we apply this to our environment, such as our home and office, we need to put in some effort to keep it tidy and organised. If we don't, disorganisation will occur spontaneously. Disorganisation has the potential to produce peak stress loads by lowering our stress tolerance, especially when it's combined with a lack of time.

Putting things you've just used straight back where they belong is an easy but powerful tool to keep your environment organised all the time. It will be neutralised as a stress inducer and will help you keep your thought processes organised too.

Sometimes we learn from opposites, so for two days, try putting everything you use back in the wrong place. Then check how your moods and stress levels are.

Don't do to be, be to be

When I first read Paul Scheele's book *Natural Brilliance*,[93] this really resonated with me. Some people try to establish their status by working at or doing something and showing it to others, or even themselves. But the idea is to be you by just being and not doing.

Let me give you an example. Staying silent within a competitive social environment and assuming appropriate body posture is often sufficient to allow you to establish a high status among the others with no need for further action.

---

93   P R Scheele, *Natural Brilliance: Overcome any challenge… at will* (Learning Strategies Corp, 2001).

Learn proper prioritisation

One of the main issues I had to contend with for many years was that I would become immersed in my first task of the day. I felt like I was being absorbed into the task like a piece of paper being sucked up by a vacuum cleaner. This allowed me to perform even small tasks with great precision, but more important tasks may have been left waiting for my attention.

Prioritise what matters most and do it first thing in the day. By focusing on the one thing that matters the most, you will progress the most. To do this, though, you will need to learn to say no to people and other tasks. Immerse yourself in the main task until it's done.

 ## Finish what you start

Nothing costs us unnecessary time and peaks our stress levels more than a job we've declared finished prematurely that we have to revisit. Even if all we have to do is to finish it, it will still come with a peak of stress loads. But the consequences may be even worse, costing us our reputation and ruining our image.

People who become bored with tasks easily and seldom finish them produce a noticeably inferior quality of work and live with the risk and fear that someone will eventually find them out. Perform all your tasks with love and dedication, and never move on without finishing them to the best of your ability. What you've done properly won't be a source of stress anymore as it will speak for your skills, reward you with a good reputation and raise your self-confidence.

Finishing a task or a project to the best of your ability raises your self-esteem and feel-good hormones and lowers your stress levels. Moving to the next task without closing the previous one will do the opposite – it will raise your cortisol levels.

Avoid multitasking

When hiring, employers are often looking for this skill in new recruits. They might want their staff to be flexible, depending on the project's priorities, but when we switch from one task to another, our productivity can go down by up to 40% each time.[94] When we are focusing on two different tasks, there are two different brain maps firing simultaneously, which makes the firing strength inefficient for both. This is especially true while we are learning. If we're multitasking, we might not be able to store the new information properly and end up not being able to recall it at all. Our recall of stored information can logically only be as

---

94 J S Rubinstein, D E Meyer and J E Evans, 'Executive control of cognitive processes in task switching' (2001), www.ncbi.nlm.nih.gov/pubmed/11518143

strong as the incoming signal when we first learned it, but not stronger.

I call multitasking 'worrying in 3D'. We have to keep track of each task, its corresponding deadline and where to take over again after the task has been on standby. The more tasks we've parked in standby mode, the more information we'll need to carry in our working memory. Consider what this does to our cortisol levels.

Focus on one task until it's completely finished, then move on. Develop this work ethic and you will get a more intense reward by finishing each task and moving to the next rather than carrying a few tasks concurrently.

Avoid accumulation

Going beyond multitasking, we want to avoid scheduling complicated tasks too close to each other, when we have the freedom to do so, to avoid overlapping and an accumulation of stress. If you need to book a dentist appointment and you have an exam coming up, for instance, schedule them a few days apart so that there is no interference between the two heavy stress loads, resulting in an accumulation of stress. Think about induced waves on a lake's surface by two epicentres. The nearer the epicentres are to each other, the higher the amplitude of the accumulated waves.

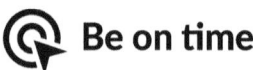 Be on time

There are three kinds of people – those who always arrive early, those who are habitually late and those who are punctual. If you belong to the second or third group, then plan systematically ahead of appointments and travelling to save you many stress peaks. Even when you are punctual, you are walking on thin ice and unnecessarily rendering your situation vulnerable. All it takes is the slightest change in the weather or traffic conditions or you forgetting something and you will be in a peak of unnecessary stress.

Work towards belonging to the first group of people. Arrive early and read a book or prepare for the meeting. This will bring your pace down, and with it your cortisol levels. Anticipate your schedule and set your alarm to leave in good time. Try it, it's a powerful technique.

Be cortisol friendly

Remember the circadian rhythm? Cortisol levels are at their highest in the morning, and then they decline until we hit a low at around midnight. We can use this important fact to keep our stress levels at bay.

As much as possible, schedule your more demanding activities, such as presentations, decisive meetings, important phone calls and heavy physical or mental work etc, in accordance with your circadian rhythm. Usually, the most demanding tasks should be done first thing in the morning and less demanding tasks afterwards.

Let's assume that we have no options other than to have a decisive meeting later in the evening. You will be stressed the whole day until the meeting occurs and at that point the stress will peak. So, your overall cortisol levels will be elevated the whole day, peaking in the evening, which leaves you counting sheep in bed unable to sleep. It is better to avoid having such cortisol inducing activities too late in the evening.

Don't forget about breaks

Don't work more than 1.5 hours without scheduling a break. The more demanding a task is, the more breaks you have to plan. I'm talking about a few minutes where you stop looking at your screen, stand up and change location, so surfing the internet doesn't count as a break. In fact, this counts as an additional stressor.

Your brain has a defined attention span and if you prolong the working windows, it will only increase stress and lower the quality of your work. Don't worry about the time you are losing for breaks as you will be more productive and less stressed by taking them. Breaks need to be regular, otherwise their effects would be equal to nil.

Stop thinking about work during your free time

The majority of people continue thinking or talking about work in their free time. Some tell their partners or friends details that should have stayed in the office. By doing this, we extend our work day and allow it to take up more time in our life, the result being that our stress levels rise and our energy levels decrease. We cannot be as productive the following day if we have been thinking about work since we left the office without having taken a real break.

I'm not referring to stress peaks resulting from disputes at work or when you have a difficult line manager etc. In these cases, you will likely feel the urge to talk to family or close friends so they can support you, give you their opinions etc. Rather, I'm talking about technical issues or ordinary discussions about work and colleagues.

One powerful rule I set for myself and clients is this: when I step out of the office door, I stop thinking about work until I come in again tomorrow. I ask my colleagues not to talk to me about work during my free time and tell them that I won't be available again until tomorrow. They may be taken aback to start with, but the majority of them understand and respect my request. Some even implement it and experience the positive impact on their productivity for themselves.

You don't have to talk about work if you give 100% at work. Put a clear dividing line between your professional and private life; don't mix the two and become one of the people who only live to work. If you do, you will be living in a stress cloud and your life will become the office.

Don't buy stress

What I mean here is to avoid anything that gets your HPA axis kicking in, whether intentionally or artificially, save for real situations. When you choose to pursue a dangerous hobby or watch horror movies, even if you think it's fun, you are still stimulating your stress response, adding to what may already be a high daily stress load. It may be entertaining for your eyes, but it's not for your body and cortisol levels.

If you have a profession that doesn't cause you any stress at all, then go ahead and watch the new *Chucky* movie. If you don't, you'd do better to avoid unnecessary stimulation of your adrenals.

Your clothes

Taking care about what we wear may sound trivial and even strange, but reducing our stressors can be compared to training athletes. If we're a thousandth of a second away from the world record, we want to optimise all parameters.

If we force ourselves to wear something we despise, perhaps something that was given to us as gift, it can be a source of considerable stress. Rather, we need to wear something which is perfectly in line with our character and the actual purpose we have for the time we're wearing it. This will free our mind and let us focus with confidence on the more important tasks of the day. The adage that clothes make people surely has some truth in it.

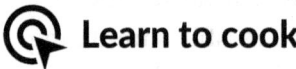 Learn to cook

Cooking can be a relaxing activity where you completely switch off to focus on your creations with their colours and flavours. It's a project for which you make a plan and put it into action. Cooking is linked to creativity, patience, passion and reward, which could be a good template for every one of your projects.

Learning to cook doesn't necessarily mean you'll have to cook every day. It's like learning a language you'll only use when you need it. But if the only thing you can do in the kitchen is burn fried eggs, then you won't find cooking particularly relaxing.

You can start by using a book of recipes to cook your favourite food, and then progress your skills to experiment with different flavours and textures. It's learning by doing. Once you start getting the hang of cooking, you'll soon adjust the recipes to your liking according to your experience.

When you have time, cooking can be an excellent tool to relax your mind and body. You can switch on a podcast while the wifi is off and enjoy the intense experience, earning the reward of a great meal that you have created.

You don't have to keep pace with your technology

We humans have invented all kinds of tools and devices to help us do things more precisely, safely and quickly. They're designed to cope with our needs as efficiently as possible, but we must be careful that we don't compete with them. We can't impose their speed on ourselves; we can't be as fast as virtual intelligence, for example. If we try, we will end up living in a stress cloud. Technology is just a tool to boost our work rate by helping us to achieve more, safely and precisely.

Virtual detox

I know a few 'dinosaurs' who refrain from using mobile phones or smartphones and they have survived so far, but unfortunately their numbers are declining. If we list all sources of stress in our lives, the use of smart devices would be likely to represent the lion's share. We tend to check our phones hundreds of times, spending a large part of each day looking at screens and forgetting that social media tools are designed to make us addicted. That's how they survive and thrive – the more they can retain our attention, the more they earn.

Every time we scroll down the timelines of our social media accounts, we get a dopamine surge which makes us want to keep on scrolling. All the colours, notifications, videos that start automatically, have been designed with the goal of surging our dopamine to keep us on the site. Dopamine is the neurotransmitter responsible for giving us the motivation and drive to accomplish things and be rewarded. If it surges too often due to a virtual trigger, we will crave more dopamine which drains our focus, energy levels and motivation. Social media addiction can be as dangerous as drug addiction.

Social media also allow our personal data to be accessible to others. They call it connectivity, but it's actually akin to new-age voyeurism. People who use their mobile phones heavily can become cold in their relationships and lose their empathy. They are hyperconnected, but lonely. Some call it digital dementia, but I call it IQ outsourcing. We have outsourced our ability for orientation to the GPS device, our ability to do maths to the calculator, our ability for organisation to our organiser app, our ability to remember to our alarm app, and that's just for starters.

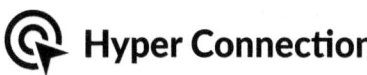 Hyper Connection

Real freedom is being able to switch your phone off for a day or two. We are connected with the world today as never before, but we are also lonelier than ever before. We can so easily end up with 2,500 fake friends who effectively leave us alone with our stress. My strategy here would be to:

- Remove all unnecessary apps, especially social media, from your smartphone. You can have them on your computer if you need them for professional reasons.

- Stop following all virtual friends with negative feeds.

- Accept friend requests only from real friends and acquaintances with whom you share at least one passion or interest.

- Schedule smart-device-free time in your week. Start with half a day and progress from there.

- Keep mobile phones on flight mode with the GPS switched off and only switch them on when you really need to use them.

- Don't subscribe to flat-rate internet access for your smartphone.

- Make it a promise if you have kids that they will never see you using your mobile phone. Many of the designers of apps will not allow their own kids to have profiles on social media.

Choose your source of information wisely

Information sources that don't come with the intention of consumer manipulation and programming are as rare as honest politicians. This is especially true for news and movies. There tends to be nothing on our screen, even in the background, that doesn't have this intention, so choose your sources of information carefully.

I banned TV from my home a decade ago, realising each time I watched the news, my mood would be at its lowest. I can't ever remember watching TV or consuming any regular media and feeling thrilled and motivated afterwards. Now I cherry pick my sources of information and follow trustworthy channels on video platforms.

Get a chauffeur

If you are a CEO, owner of a big business or someone with a lot of responsibility, this technique is for you. Your free time for relaxation is tight, you work to schedule and can only give your attention to the highest priorities. Delegation becomes a necessity and driving should not be an exception, even if you love to drive.

I'm sure I'm not alone in loving to drive on the open road, but driving around cities or on congested roads can be a major stress inducer, especially if it's combined with tight schedules. Getting a chauffeur will allow you to reduce your stress input by sitting back and ignoring the traffic while travelling. You can then read or listen to a podcast or do a last review prior to a meeting.

These are some techniques to reduce your lifestyle stress right away, but what about for the long term? That's exactly what we're going to look at next.

10
Mastering Lifestyle Stress – Long-term Wins

'The only sure way to avoid making mistakes is to have no new ideas.'
— Albert Einstein

Embrace failure

'All great things come after failure'
— Justin Williams

Never focus on success alone, otherwise your fall will be steep. Of course, we all work to succeed and avoid mistakes, but failure is not as evil or as bad as we may think. A ground-shaking failure is an excellent teacher.

Failure immunises us and makes us stronger for the time ahead. It makes us experienced and better at doing what we have just failed in. I personally prefer to learn from people who have gained their experience from their failures rather than success. Failure is a good antidote for arrogance as it brings us nearer to wisdom than success does. It makes us think and encourages us to be more creative, while success makes us happy for the short term, and then comes the fall with all the stress, responsibilities and changes that come with it.

If we compare it to nutrition, failure is like the good fats that support the whole body, brain and heart with sustained energy, and success is like carbohydrates which make us happy for the short term, but after spiking our insulin, they cause us to crash. And if you believe that fat is evil, then let me tell you that cholesterol becomes even worse after glycation by glucose.

In this age of smart devices, many of us seem to be focused on success without failing, so we need to rethink on our relationship with failure. Failure and success are two sides of the same coin. Neutralise your fear of and stress load from failure by embracing it as the greatest teacher you'll ever had. When you fail, you grow by learning how not to do things. When you succeed, you grow to learn how to do things. In other words, you have more potential to learn from failing than from succeeding.

Take care of yourself

It sounds logical, but if we take care of ourselves, it will positively influence our stress levels and the way we deal with people and stress loads. But some character types may neglect themselves to please others.

Always take time to care for yourself and your wellbeing before caring about others. You can't really take care of others if you are not well. For example, eating on the go or while looking at a screen is a manifestation of self-disrespect. If we light a candle and take time to sit down with loved ones to have dinner, our hormonal responses, food absorption and the effects the food has on us are incomparably better than those of someone who's standing up and pinching bites while speaking on the phone.

Sense when you have got to take a break

Sometimes the worst thing we can do is to rush into making a decision, thinking the case is then closed. Nothing costs us more time and frustration than a bad decision made in haste, and this is especially true if it is linked to financial or irreversible loss. Nobody can quantify all the time and wealth people have lost in just one year because they have made decisions too hastily. A fraction of the combined losses could have solved a fair portion of the world's problems.

Ask yourself if it makes sense to take a bit more time or distance yourself from the issues before making a decision. Perhaps even take a break or get a couple of good nights' sleep, and then rethink your strategy again. This is especially true for important decisions which may impact others or bring about irreversible results. Try it the next time you are about to make an important decision. Prepare your decision, but don't announce it. A day or two later, go over it again and check whether your opinion is unchanged or if you see new aspects that may alter it.

Sense when to take a task by storm

There are some rules which seem to be universal. One example is a technique people regularly use during exams. Because of the density of the questions and the limited time, they start by answering the easiest questions first, and then progress on to the more difficult ones.

As rule of thumb, if you have an answer within 10 seconds, answer that question first, but if you need more time then move on to the next question. In this way, you'll finish about a third to half of the questions within the first 20% or so of the time, which will skyrocket your confidence. Unconsciously, you will be crystallising your answers for the more difficult questions, and so you'll progress step by step, doing the hardest questions at the end without pushing the time boundary.

In your professional life, you may not be as time-limited as you are during an exam, so you may tend to do the opposite. You may attack a heavyweight problem as soon as it confronts you. The main reason for this is to see it as a challenge right at the beginning with a surge of cortisol, as is the case in a fight-or-flight situation, and avoid letting it lapse to act as a continuous stressor. After the big issue is solved, you get a surge of dopamine and are more than ready to storm the rest of the tasks. This technique allows you to minimise your stress response, whether your timeframe is limited or not.

Schedule work around holidays

I learned this technique from one of my mentors. When he schedules the year ahead, he starts with his holidays first, and then fits work around them. In this way, he has been able to dramatically lower his stress levels and make even more money than before with about 10% of his former team.

Schedule your holidays at the end of December for the year to come. If you don't have kids, exclude school holidays. Once that's done, fill the gaps with milestones for your targeted achievements.

Sport is a stressor

Sporting activity is more important for us than it was for our ancestors. They used their bodies as they were designed to be used and didn't need to perform sports or go to the gym to maintain their health and strength.

Aerobic activities, for example jogging or cycling, have an undeniable positive impact on cardiovascular health, but they primarily impact the stress hormone with no noticeable impact on androgens, testosterone and GH. If you do them on a long-term basis, they will ensure you have higher cortisol levels, which in turn ensures your body will consume your muscle mass to supply amino acids and store fat as soon as it starts feeding on itself. If you push your body to the extreme, like training for a marathon, the body consumes all it can. Relate this to a pro marathon runner and compare his or her strength and muscle mass to a sprinter.

Remember, your best ally against aging is your muscle mass. It sounds extreme, but excessive cardio is like stepping on the accelerator when the car is going downhill. With age, your body will get rid of unnecessary muscle mass anyway because of the wrong signal being sent to the brain. If you don't use your muscles properly, the body will reduce its muscle mass to adapt to your real daily needs.

Let's have a quick look at a premium tool used by all athletes: strength training. Strength training, when it's done properly, will benefit your androgens tremendously. Even if your cortisol rises during the session, the androgens will mask its negative effects.

You don't have to train indoors if you prefer being outdoors. There are gyms with outside areas for modified strongmen (MST) training, which is great fun and highly effective for fat loss and conditioning. It is normally done in groups.

Let's list the progressions to convert from steady state cardio:

1. Minimise cardio and limit it to a maximum of one hour per session and not more than twice a week. By doing this, you will keep your cortisol release low. Longer lasting aerobic efforts produce more cortisol in relation to testosterone and create a catabolic environment in the long run. Studies have shown the adverse effects of longer lasting aerobic efforts on the testosterone to cortisol ratio.[95][96][97]

---

[95] Ahmad H Alghadir, Sami A Gabr and Farag A Aly, 'The effects of four weeks aerobic training on saliva cortisol and testosterone in young healthy persons' (2015), www.ncbi.nlm.nih.gov/pmc/articles/PMC4540811/

[96] G Banfi et al., 'Usefulness of free testosterone/cortisol ratio during a season of elite speed skating athletes' (1993), www.ncbi.nlm.nih.gov/pubmed/8244603/

[97] G Lutoslawska et al., 'Plasma cortisol and testosterone following 19-km and 42-km kayak races' (1991), www.ncbi.nlm.nih.gov/pubmed/1806731

2. Walk outdoors for one or more hours many times during the week. Such a low intensity steady state (LISS) exercise as walking has no real impact on cortisol or androgens but has an increased positive affect and a reduced negative affect. Best results were shown when walking in nature or/and with a good company.[98] Walking goes extremely well with listening to a podcast or an audiobook.

3. Do high-intensity interval training (HIIT) sprints if you can. If you would struggle with these then there are other HIIT options that can be done as on an air resistance exercise bike or while swimming. HIIT, in a similar way to strength training, impacts on cortisol and androgens. It is also timesaving. Usually you do between 20 and 40 minutes, which includes warming up. You can do HIIT while climbing or boxing, so it never gets boring. HIIT also has an after-burner effect and can burn body fat for a long time, especially for new trainees.[99]

4. The next progression would be strength training with the option of MST if you like being outdoors. This is the most effective tool for shedding fat, getting stronger and positively impacting your hormonal and neurotransmitter profiles.

---

[98] Marcus Johansson, Terry Hartig and Henk Staats, 'Psychological benefits of walking: moderation by company and outdoor environment' (2011), www.researchgate.net/publication/229975327

[99] E Borsheim and R Bahr, 'Effect of exercise intensity, duration and mode on post-exercise oxygen consumption' (2003), www.ncbi.nlm.nih.gov/pubmed/14599232

You will absolutely need an amino acid shake during your workout. This will keep your cortisol level under control and save your muscle mass from being catabolised.

Overtraining

Overtraining happens if the balance between effort and recovery is disturbed, possibly due to an increase in frequency, volume or load of the training sessions, or poor recovery. All elements of stress management – sleep quality, nutrition etc – play a role in whether we overtrain and how quickly we can rectify matters.

When we overtrain, our strength, cognitive function, attention span and, of course, stress tolerance levels all drop. The only thing which goes up is the risk of injury. If we're on a calorie-deficit or carb-free diet, we're likely to overtrain more easily than if we're on a calorie-surplus diet or one that includes carbs. The risk of overtraining also correlates to age – the older we are, the easier it is to overtrain.

ANDRE'S STORY

My mentor, Andre Benoit, knows how to tell a story about overtraining from his time preparing for the 1992 Winter Olympics in Albertville as a member of the Canadian luge team. Charles R Poliquin, who was the strength coach of the Canadian team, had put the team on an intensification phase. They pushed each other through crushing workouts and, since they were lifting maximum weights very close to their respective one rep maximum, their central nervous system fatigued further with each training session. After four weeks Charles came back to the training camp and noticed that everyone's hands were trembling. When he realised that this 'Parkinson'-like trembling had been present for a few days already, he immediately ordered all athletes to have four days completely off as this was a sign that the team had over trained the CNS and needed some rest. This is to say that there are multiple parameters which have a direct impact on your performance and the ability to recover.

But don't take overtraining too seriously, though. There are people who use it as an excuse to skip going to the gym, but the absolute majority of us train within our comfort zone and don't know the rules of diminishing return or progressive overload. We remain loyal to our exercise routine and see no results after the first two weeks. If we want results then we need to go out of the comfort zone as nothing grows in it but be aware to not over train. It's a sailing between both limits.

As a rule of thumb, I would say if you are younger than forty, then you can train five times a week or more, as long as you sleep for 8 hours each night, without risking overtraining. The sweet spot is four sessions per week, but if you want faster progression, five sessions per week will be great. And this doesn't mean you can't do more. If you are a gym fanatic who wants to boost your progress, mass or strength, then one of the best methods is to increase your training frequency to twice per day. But as with everything, you must manage recovery and nutrition on a pro-level.

If you are over forty, the rule of thumb would be to train for two days and then schedule one or two days off, if you want to be on the safe side. Listen to your body, it talks to you non-stop.

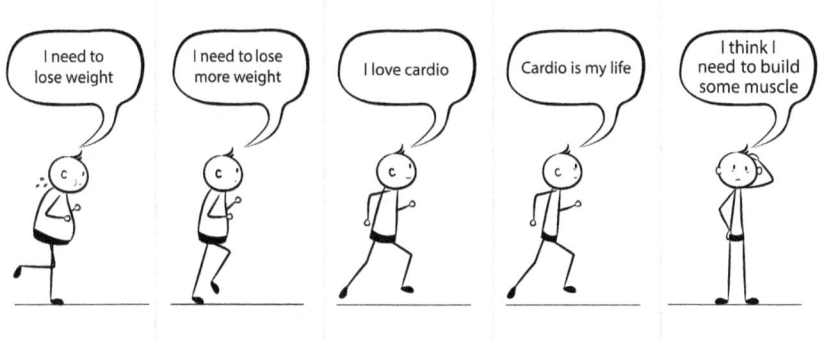

Be minimalistic

Since we humans stopped being nomads and settled down, we have been accumulating things, but storing stuff we don't really need clutters up our brain, in particular our memory, with the things we are not using. The more we accumulate, the more our brain will be unnecessarily busy keeping track of everything.

Imagine you are on a long journey. The more unnecessary things you carry with you, the more you'll be burdened by luggage. Be minimalistic in your way of life and keep your brain ready to think and create. Don't use it as storage space for things you don't use.

Don't swim against the flow

Sometimes everything in life seems to be going against us and loading us with stress triggers, which can come simultaneously or consecutively. There are so many stress triggers that we feel totally overwhelmed and overrun by them. At these times, the best way to deal with the stressors may not be to fight against them, but rather swim along with them. Otherwise, we may risk burning out while trying to manage the entire stress load at the same time.

Let yourself go – go on a recovery retreat, have a massage or sauna, or do something entirely new to you. Ideally, it would be something which is fun and makes you laugh, helping to erase the memory of the stress triggers. Often, when you are on a retreat, time will work wonders and a few of the stress triggers will vanish as quickly as they arrived, motivating you to solve the remaining ones.

NICK'S CASE

Two years prior to hiring me as his coach, Nick was knocking at obesity's door. He weighed 95 kg (210 lbs) with a height of 1.78 m (5 foot 10). Then he found a passion for sports and shed his body fat to build an athletic body. He was swimming up to 3 km, playing badminton for hours and cycling about 70 km on weekends. This was what he had been doing for two years until he hired me.

When we started working together, he was weighing in at 54 kg and looked really weak. With his type of training, he had burnt more than 40 kg of his body weight. The common denominator of all his activity choices was that they were aerobic. What had started as motivation to get healthy, shed body fat and gain his dream physique ended in chronically elevated cortisol levels, which had burnt fat and muscle mass, and probably bone too.[100]

After conducting the initial interview and the Hormonal Profile Assessment, I was sure my main working lever in the first weeks with Nick would primarily be cortisol. The first priority was to manage his cortisol levels to a healthy circadian rhythm by minimising stress input while helping him increase his sleep quality and length. The most important step was for him to have a distinct break from what he was doing to give him enough time to recover from the training. I taught him how to do this by minimising exposure to stressors like electronic displays, EMF and to make use of earthing, such as walking barefoot in the garden or at the beach, and

---

100 E Canalis and A M Delany, 'Mechanisms of glucocorticoid action in bone' (2002), www.ncbi.nlm.nih.gov/pubmed/12114261

sunlight to reset his system, priorities and circadian rhythm. Starting a demanding training programme without marking a clear break from his previous exercise routine would have stressed him even further without showing any results.

When I revealed my strategy for the first month to him, he was shocked. Imagine how someone who has been doing sports daily for two years would feel at being asked to stop them all for two to three weeks; he wasn't expecting this as he thought he'd hired a coach to train him and it was hard for him to accept. He came up with suggestions like 'Can't I keep the volume low or just stretch?' but I wasn't willing to give up on my primary lever.

A few days later, Nick was starting to increase his sleep length and quality. After just one week, he was sleeping regularly for 8 hours. After two weeks, we started with training. He was fresh and motivated like the falcon.

Four weeks in, Nick had regained 5 kg of his body weight, most of it muscle. After 9 months of training, Nick had gained about 12 kg of mass (9.5 kg lean mass) and massively increased his strength for all exercises. His focus had gone up, he was feeling healthy and his body was functioning well again.

11
Mastering Social Stress – Immediate Wins

'Before you speak, let your words pass through three gates:
Is it true?
Is it necessary?
Is it kind?'
— Rumi

One of the more interesting studies on social stress is from Holmes and Rahe.[101] They identified common life events and gave them a score depending on their severity as a stress trigger. The total score of recent events gives a person's probability of illness in the next two years.

---

[101] TH Holmes and RH Rahe, 'The social readjustment rating scale,' *Journal of Psychosomatic Research*, 11/2 (1967), 213–218

We are hugely influenced by our social field, especially in terms of it acting as a source of stress. This is one of the biggest parts of our stress input, so we need to master it by working on ourselves or on the stress emitters. We will see from the techniques shared in this chapter and the next how all these stress sources can become easily manageable.

Smile

Activating both of your zygomaticus major muscles, which are the main muscles you use to smile, has a huge impact on your brain and stress response. Even if you don't have a reason for smiling, regularly activating those muscles will make sure you keep your stress load low by releasing feel-good neurotransmitters such as dopamine and serotonin.[102] This is a chemical response of the nervous system to a true smile. Smiling is free, easy to do, intense and says more than a thousand lines of poetry.

Smiling is one of my strengths. I can't say good morning to someone without accompanying it with a smile, so I don't have direct experience of having to learn how to do it, but if I had to learn it, I would recall a funny situation or time spent with a good friend.

---

102 R D Lane, 'Neural Correlates of Conscious Emotional Experience', in RD Lane and L Nadel (eds) *Cognitive Neuroscience of Emotion* (Oxford University Press, 2000), pp. 345–370.

Smiling is the best trust and friendship builder. It signals that you are interested in building bridges with the person in front of you, that you don't have anything against them, that you respect them and that they are important to you. A smile connects you with others who want to walk the same walk. It's the most beautiful way to offer your friendship to someone. Smiling will impact people in your surroundings and spread positive vibes, which will help to keep their stress input low.

Unfortunately, there are people who see smiling as a weakness and may look at you with disdain, or in extreme cases even want to harm you. Beware of them. Don't give them the blink of an eye of a chance to do this, but don't forget to keep smiling.

Greeting

Greeting is the key to communication, and communication is the key to understanding. This doesn't mean that we won't or can't communicate without a greeting, but we are more likely to have easy communication with someone we greet than with someone we don't greet.

Greeting, in a similar way to a smile, is an offer of friendship, which is free. And not greeting does exactly the opposite. It unwittingly communicates that the person we're addressing isn't important to us, they're in some way inferior and/or we don't actually like or need them in our life.

One step on from greeting is greeting+. If we're greeting someone, we have three ways of doing it. We reply to their greeting with the same enthusiasm they have shown if we want to give a sense of importance to them which is just right, but not too much. Greeting them with less enthusiasm than they have shown could demonstrate that they're someone we don't want to deal with any longer. And if we greet them with more love and enthusiasm than they have shown to us, it indicates they are someone we would like to extend our friendship and connection with.

We tend to do this unintentionally anyway. The rule here is that if we want to have less stress from the people in our social circles, we should greet them with a level of enthusiasm similar to or higher than the way they greet us. This reduces their stress input on us, so even if they are hostile towards us, our greeting+ could make them rethink their strategies and become friendlier. Who knows? Managing our stress levels is all about minimising the risks of stress inputs in general, and this is a powerful tool to do just that.

Perception

A huge amount of stress when we're dealing with others is based on misunderstandings. This kind of stress is totally unnecessary and easily avoidable. We want to pay attention to how we're perceived by our social environment. It's not about how we say things, but rather how our social circle perceives our input.

Way too often, people make premature conclusions based on feelings and not facts. Make sure the people you socialise with have understood your point or request well by cross checking and questioning them. Even the smallest misunderstanding may lead to a stress load and waste your time.

Choose face-to-face or phone interactions instead of written communications. We are used to seeing, feeling and noticing every way someone else communicates, such as inflections of the voice and facial expressions. Written communications, more often than not, are liable to miss important information. We can't tell exactly how they're meant – whether the communicator is angry or joking, for example – which opens the door to misinterpretation.

Be clear, short and friendly, and keep certain discussions for face-to-face encounters. Don't give people any chance to go against you and create unnecessary stress loads based on misinterpretations.

Reconfirm

Often mistakes happen in professional life because of weak communication leading to a misunderstanding between the two parties. A powerful tool to mitigate this risk – a tool I have adopted for many years which has been proven to be 100% reliable – is a final confirmation between the partners involved in the communication. At the end of a discussion, ask questions about the key points and let the other parties confirm them, showing that they have really understood them.

Sometimes you need written confirmation if you are dealing with a client or a difficult relationship. In these cases, keep a red line of proof and let them confirm it in written form. By reconfirming everything for total clarity, I have been able to massively reduce stress and the potential for miscommunication that can negatively impact the team and the working atmosphere.

Be kind(er)

I'm not implying that you aren't putting in the effort to work on your performance as I'm quite sure you are, but the busy lifestyle we all lead and the electronics and gadgets we use almost constantly can work against us and make us forget about kindness and the moments we should dedicate to others. Kindness and readiness to help others reflect on our personality. It's like a mirror where we get to see what we put in front of it.

Ideally, greet and talk to everyone, including people outside your social or competence levels, in exactly the same way as you would talk to your boss. Kindness shouldn't be dependent on who's receiving it; it should be dependent on the source, which is your heart. Use the same smile, same enthusiasm and same level of kindness for the boss and the cleaner.

If you're dealing with someone, then they are worthy of kindness, and if they don't respond in a similar way, the stress loads they pass on to you will be low and you'll feel strong because you didn't stoop to their level.

Give without expecting

Don't expect anything in return when you're giving, whether it's kindness or anything else, at least not from the one you're giving to. Doing otherwise will open you up to waiting, and waiting is dependency, and dependency makes you weak and can be a source of stress.

Never compare yourself to others

Never compare yourself with people in a negative way, for example in regard to how much they have or earn. You are yourself, no one else. How much you or other people own isn't important; it's all about how effective you, and they, are at dealing with it.

You can compare yourself of today with the you of yesterday and define what the you of tomorrow should be. Set targets for yourself and regularly ask questions about what you have achieved in the timeframe you've set for your goals. What have you learned? How have you progressed? Which goals are you still focusing on? Set them as targets for the next steps.

Never promise

Avoid promising as much as possible. Besides ringing the bells of unprofessionalism, a promise potentially creates unnecessary stress loads. It's like a minefield that could explode anywhere and everywhere.

Let's adopt a probability approach here. If you have made 5,000 promises in your life, do you truly believe you can or will honour them all and always deliver on time? Even if you are good, you may miss a few hundred promises, and that's enough damage done.

Forget about the minesweeper game of promises. In real life, there is no smiley reset button.

🎯 Power hug

When I feel down or need a boost, I ask my kids to give me a big hug each. A sincere hug from a loved one can decrease stress levels and increase feel-good hormones instantaneously.

Being connected to people we love has an impact on a hormone called oxytocin. Oxytocin, which is released by the posterior pituitary gland, is known as a female hormone as it's a facilitator for birth and lactation, but it seems to have far-reaching effects on the wellbeing of us all. I remember when my wife gave birth to our first son, I had a painful migraine in sync with her pains. I asked her once the baby had found his way to her breast if she could imagine ever giving birth and going through all the pain again, and she said yes. That shows how powerful oxytocin, also known as the love hormone, is.

Besides promoting mother-and-child bonding, attachment and improvement of social skills, oxytocin has a suppressing effect on cortisol by modulating the HPA axis and regulating functions of the autonomic nervous system.[103] The love hormone even has anti-inflammatory properties as it decreases oxidation and releases pro-inflammatory cytokines.[104]

---

[103] C S Carter, 'Neuroendocrine perspectives on social attachment and love' (1998), www.ncbi.nlm.nih.gov/pubmed/9924738

[104] A Szeto et al., 'Oxytocin attenuates NADPH-dependent superoxide activity and IL-6 secretion in macrophages and vascular cells' (2008), www.ncbi.nlm.nih.gov/pubmed/18940936

Dr S Carter, who has extensively researched the far-reaching effects of the love hormone, highlights that oxytocin can facilitate adult neurogenesis and tissue repair, especially after a stressful experience.[105] Exposure to oxytocin early in life seems to have a huge impact not only on our ability to love and form social bonds as adults, but also on our health and wellbeing in general, hence the importance of regular hugs and physical contact with your kids. It ingrains in them a sense of love and compassion for now and years to come.

Rely on nobody but yourself

Relying on others makes you dependent on them, and dependency keeps you waiting, hoping, anticipating and guessing. It kills your motivation, disturbs your schedule and makes you vulnerable to stress and anxiety. Avoid relying on others as much as you can, and if you absolutely have to rely on someone, have a backup plan. Don't wait. Remember, no one else has your success at heart other than you.

Look for solutions not accusations

If you want to reduce the stress that can be induced by conflicts, you have to be serious about looking for

---

105 C Sue Carter and Stephen W Porges, 'The biochemistry of love: an oxytocin hypothesis' (2013), www.ncbi.nlm.nih.gov/pmc/articles/PMC3537144/

solutions and not take the road of accusations. Accusations are a one-way street leading to a dead end. Even if they know they are wrong, few people will admit it. Accusations have the potential to go into overdrive and produce peak stress inputs. Be the neutral problem-solver, even if you are not neutral, and don't lose your focus on the solution. It's the white rabbit, so chase it.

You don't have to convince

If you are convinced about something and believe in it, you may like others to experience the same conviction. You may then tend to make a huge effort to convince others, especially if they don't share the same ideas or views as you, but doing this carries the potential for stress generation. Other people may not experience the same conviction and could make you responsible for their bad choices. Instead of convincing people, explain and describe your experience, but always add a disclaimer to cover yourself.

Mind love

Being able to love is a gift in itself, but as much as it can be a source of happiness in life, it can also be as bitter as death. It's just about being careful; no one would blame car manufacturers for including airbags in cars because of the extra weight.

Know that everyone in your life will leave one day, regardless of how close, vulnerable or dependent they are now. They will find their reasons to do so, so love, but never be dependent. Leave some neurons to cope with the worst case scenario. Be independent enough to relaunch a new life when there is no other way out.

Avoid being dependent

It's crucial to have good connections, whether with your relatives and friends, or you're networking for business and developmental reasons, but never become dependent on anyone, regardless of how close or reliable they are. It doesn't have to do with trust – I guess you have already proof-checked them if you've let them come into your life – but no one knows when they may leave for good.

Avoid toxic people

Negative people are like black holes. They suck you into their lives and beat you up with all their problems. You, as a problem-solver, will give them potential solutions, but I've never met a toxic person who's genuinely interested in solving their issues. They just want to keep you busy by offering you an extensive insight into their trash; they're are not going to implement any of your solutions.

Don't play their game. Identify toxic people and avoid them at all costs. Protect your motivation, time and cortisol levels. Just flee! Similarly, and excuse the profanity, avoid dick-headed people. If someone prefers to argue rather than listen and learn, this is an indicator that you should flee from them too.

Take time to judge

Don't judge and jump to hasty conclusions. You never know what someone's actual reason is for their behaviour. Extend enough time to clarify and understand situations fully, and build a reserve of excuses for your friends, family and partners. You can gauge if their behaviour is in harmony with their character, and often there are other reasons behind their actions which are hidden from you. Don't aggravate the situation and risk losing their trust by being judgmental based on flimsy evidence.

Honour your decisions

Once you have carefully made a decision based on facts, stick to it and don't question it. Questioning your decisions risks frustration and stress loads and is a black hole, swallowing your time. This doesn't mean you shouldn't be flexible enough to modify your decision; you always need a back door, but only if the circumstances have changed.

Don't ask for things you don't like to be asked for

Prior to asking for things, question whether you would like to be asked for the same. If your answer is no or maybe, then move on and do it yourself.

Let's take an example. Some people tend to ask their friends and family for financial help. This isn't a bad request per se, but no one really likes to be asked that question, especially if the money is for trivial things.

Questioning whether you would want to be asked for the thing you're planning to ask someone else for will save your friendships and reputation. No one likes to be around people who take advantage of their friends.

These are some of the most effective ways to manage social stress that I have come across, and you can put them into action immediately. In the next chapter, we will look at some equally effective long-term wins for gaining control over this type of stress.

12
Mastering Social Stress – Long-term Wins

'A good way to overcome stress is to help others out of theirs.'
— Dada J P Vaswani

Social circle and the solar system

One of my closest friends once told me that people are like planets. Planets have their defined trajectory in space, and if they come within a split of a hair nearer to the sun, they collide with each other. And if they go the same infinitesimal distance further away, they drift from the solar system.

The way this translates into real life is that there are people you can see every day without them being a source of stress, and there are others you'd be better off seeing only once in a while. Every relationship needs its own trajectory to function properly. Were you to force it to change, you would lose it. But it's going to be a game of trial and error until you find the right distance.

Build your tribe

Try to create your own tribe with a group of people who might need your mental or financial support, knowledge or encouragement in hard times in order to help them grow and avoid unnecessary mistakes in their lives. They might be younger than you, at least in terms of experience, and therefore might need someone who can give them the right advice and lead them. Invest time and gather the right people around you. If you have chosen your tribe carefully, they will speak for your generosity, support you and defend you when need be.

Have brothers and sisters

I call these people gatekeepers. They are the people who know you and you know them better than anyone else. Your gatekeepers can become closer to you than your own brothers and sisters as you can choose them; they aren't just fair-weather friends. You know they'll be there when you need them. In trying times, they will be the ones sharing your pain and giving their support and sincere advice. Having just one gatekeeper is far more beneficial and rewarding than having thousands of fake friends.

Share your pains with your gatekeepers. Talk to them, as they will support you honestly with subjective decisions and dare to tell you when you are in the wrong. They will help you recognise the wood from the trees.

Just as Rome wasn't built in a day, you won't form these close ties overnight. You need to nurture and grow them like a tree that needs years of care to bear fruit. Start taking care of your garden now if you don't wish to sit in the middle of a dry, barren land later on.

Children

If you are single, your stress is one-fold; if you're married, then your stress is multi-fold; but if you have children, your stress is huge, depending on the number you have and which genes are being activated. If you master this stress Shaolin monks will come to seek advice from you.

Children, as stress emitters, cannot be compared to other people in our social environment. Stress loads coming from them can be highly amplified as we are closely emotionally tied to them. As parents, we are sensitive and receptive, and so are vulnerable to this kind of stress.

It's similar to hormone sensitivity. When you are resistant, even high hormone secretions may not be able to pass on the message; when you are sensitive, small hormone releases will be sufficient. Your receptors are wide awake and waiting for even the weakest signals. That's how it is when you have children.

> 'A head won't grow until another becomes grey.'
> — Algerian proverb

If you love your living space to be tidy at all times, with children you will have to embrace chaos. If you have daily rituals such as drinking a coffee in the morning, writing your diary or enjoying a good book, accept and expect them to be interrupted. A short article may take you days to read. Children decide on your schedule, day and night, and your life's not your own anymore. You will only have free time for yourself when they are asleep or in school.

Welcome to flexible organisation!

I love my kids beyond everything. Children are the greatest of gifts, and at the same time the biggest responsibility we can have. They are like a blank book in which we can write whatever we want, but once it's written, there is no going back, and therein lies the big responsibility. Their future depends on us. We can teach them to become great or not so great. Bringing up children well is a chance for us to give something back to the community and influence the world for the good. If we have written their books well, then we have hope that our children will one day be there for us when we need them.

With children, there are different kinds of stress loads depending on the phase they are in. It starts prior to their birth with all the pains of pregnancy, and then the postpartum stage with the sleepless nights and baby blues, and the list goes on and on. Everything related to their health, wellbeing and future keeps us busy and worried. We never stop, even when they are grown up and independent. They will always have a special bond with us which keeps us thinking about them.

But kids don't only come with stress loads. The beauty is their positive impact on us. Just a hug, a look or a touch can improve our mood tremendously and instantaneously. Seeing them growing up and progressing on a daily basis is a stress remedy.

Coincidentally, while I was writing those lines, my daughter came along and asked if I needed a hug. When I said of course I did, she asked why and I told her that her hug would give me good ideas to continue writing. She then gave me a big hug. Her brother heard the discussion and didn't want to be excluded, so he came running over and gave me a hug too.

There is no way to bypass the stress load having kids involves other than to work on ourselves by establishing a strong and balanced outlook on life. If they feel that we are weak, our children will feel insecure and will be afraid to develop and grow. We need to give them confidence in themselves and teach them self-respect, respect for others and for nature, and how they can be successful by using their brains and physicality. For this, we need to be prepared with techniques to apply and be ready to learn and grow with them.

In terms of patience, I can definitely say my kids are the best teachers. They push me to my limits, but I lose the fight if I start thinking and acting as a busy adult who is not living in the moment. They have taught me to live in the present when I'm with them.

Children grow quickly. The stages of their development succeed one another in a flash and are irreversible. Enjoy each moment as intensely as you can as this is the only way not to have regrets later on.

Your kids' stress

Whether we like it or not, the biggest challenge we're likely to face while bringing up children in the modern world is to reduce their access to electronic displays and smart devices. At home, my family has one iMac, two MacBook Pros, two iPads, two iPhones, one tablet and one Kindle, so our house looks like a tech store. The kids used to have access to iPads, iPhones and sometimes my wife's MacBook Pro to watch movies on, but when we became aware how dangerous EMF radiation, blue light and dopamine addiction are for them, we gradually reduced their exposure. Here's how we did it:

- We explained the risks and showed them videos about how dangerous this exposure can be for them.

- Once they understood the dangers, we offered to do a deal with them to reduce their consumption to just games and educational apps, without the need for wifi use, and a maximum of one movie per week. The movies are downloaded while they are at school and they always have to make sure the flight mode is on if they are using the iPads or iPhones and the screen is on nightshift mode, even during the day, so as not to disturb their circadian rhythms.

- A few weeks later, we made the iPads and iPhones disappear and left them with just the MacBook Pro for their one movie per week, and that's where they are right now.

Of course, the children ask for the iPads and iPhones from time to time, but when I remind them how dangerous they are for them, they quickly give up. Start this process as soon as possible with your kids, as the longer they use technology, the harder it will become for them to give it up.

Here are a few more ways we keep our kids' stress levels low:

- We hug them regularly, especially when they wake up and go to bed. They need plenty of love and physical contact, even more than adults, to acquire confidence and recharge.
- We talk to them as equals to gain their trust.
- We think carefully prior to making decisions, but once we've made the decision, we stick to it. Any exceptions have to be fully justifiable to the kids.
- We use their short attention span to switch discussions on to good topics.
- We realise they copy every detail from us, so we're aware of everything we want to write in their book.
- We use pre-notices. For example, we will say, 'In 5 minutes we will leave the playground', and then 5 minutes later, 'Time is up, let's go'. This is much better than springing 'Now we go home, finished' on them.
- We make sure they have regular energy release opportunities in the form of playing outdoors.
- We motivate them to do sports, encouraging them to try as many sports as they can from as early an

age as possible so they can choose the right ones. This is quite important as coordination stagnates around the age of 12.

- We don't force them to do the things we like or would like them to do. Instead, we help them understand all the options and make the right decision based on facts and awareness.

In terms of general stress management with the kids, we have found it works wonders to record their misdemeanours on score cards, and if they reach five in one day, then they are not allowed to go out the day after. In such stressful situations, they start counting their points and debating who has fewer, and the stress is changed to a game to test their memory and maths. They can also reduce their points by doing good things, so they keep motivated to make up for a mistake to reduce their score and increase their chances of being allowed out the next day.

Should you, from time to time, be overwhelmed by a situation and lose a fight with your kids, just let it pass and calm down. A child's ability to forget and forgive works wonders. Later come back for a review and assessment of your reaction and identify the root cause, then come up with a strategy to avoid the point of divergence in the future and add it to your toolbox. The more you learn from such situations, the more immunised to this type of stress you and your kids will become. Remember, you will always get to read back over what you have written in your book.

Be yourself

It sounds bizarre, but often people don't know themselves. This may be because their focus is on external factors or material things, or due to the fact that they have never thought they might not know themselves. Know yourself by studying your nature, strengths, capabilities, capacities, limiting factors and weaknesses.

If you don't know yourself well enough, you may fall into the trap of trying to be someone else. Trying to be someone else is energy sapping and will get you nowhere. Being yourself is more natural, it won't require extra energy, plus it makes you more consistent and balances you in life. It makes you original and gets you the right friends.

Care less about others' opinions

There is an Arabian anecdote which shows what happens to people who are too receptive to the opinions of others. Juha, an old man, had a young son and a donkey, which he wanted to sell. He decided to ask his son to accompany him to the city's Friday market.

On the way, they decided to walk beside their donkey until they met a group of people. The people regarded them and said, 'Look at them. They have a donkey and they don't even ride it. How dumb are they?'

Juha decided to let his son ride on the donkey until they met the next group of people. These people looked at them and said, 'What a spoilt boy. His father walks while he is riding on the donkey.'

Juha then decided to ride the donkey himself and let his son walk, until they met the next group of people. They said, 'What a cruel father, making his young son walk while he is riding the donkey.'

With that in mind, Juha and his son both got on to the donkey. But the next group of people they met said, 'What a cruel family! They have no mercy for the poor animal.'

When Juha heard this, he said to his son, 'Go pick up the donkey's front feet, I will pick up the rear feet, and we'll carry him. Then I won't worry about the opinions of others again.'

The moral here is if you try to make everyone around you happy, you will keep yourself busy and unhappy.

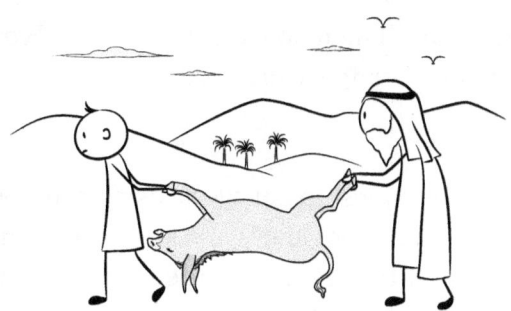

Contact with officials

There are people who stress out and get into anxiety mode when they come into contact with officials like the police, government agents etc. If you are one, realise that you are dealing with mere humans. They eat, drink and sleep, and they may even have the same fear of other officials as you have of them.

See the processes behind official people rather than regarding them as people with too much power and help them perform their job well. Often, it helps lower your anxiety to put yourself in their shoes and ask yourself how you would feel in their position. See 'Tune your heart in to coherence' in Chapter 7 to remind yourself how to influence people in a positive direction.

Colleagues and lakes

Your work may be the source of major stress in your life. This is likely to be due to bad relationships with colleagues and line managers, which may even stray into bullying, or the work itself not being right for you.

I think of relationships at work using the lines that measure the different levels of a lake. Those lines represent several thresholds in order to assess the state of a lake, and one is the line of no return. As long as the level of the water is above this line, the lake can regenerate itself from rain or ground sources. But if the water level falls below the line of no return, then drought is inevitable. It's just a matter of time.

You need to invest in your job to keep relationships in a healthy state, but you also need to sense when you've crossed the line of no return, and you'd be better off leaving before this happens. If you don't, you'll create a massive stress load which may grey your hair while you're losing your most precious resource: time.

Invest in good relationships

Relationships are like plants. If you neglect or mistreat them, they will die. If you have a healthy relationship with someone, you'll feel that it's strong and reliable, but to get to this point, it will have to survive a few tests and challenges to nurture and develop it, so invest in worthy relationships and get rid of draining ones.

Don't speak negatively of others

The best among us are the ones who are preoccupied with our own matters and don't waste time on the matters of others. This extends to talking and thinking about others, except if it is to learn from their successes or failures, as it is a total waste of time. It keeps you busy doing nothing and kills the most precious resource of all: time. Gossiping about others pulls you down like a hot-air balloon with a gaping hole in it. You can't have a positive mindset while you are talking negatively about others, even if it's true. The two don't and can't function together.

Don't spread the bad word

In a similar way, moaning about conflicts or bad experiences you have had may make you feel better for a short time, but it is likely to bring you and your entire social circle down in the long term. If you need to talk about something you have been through, speak with your gatekeepers, the brothers and sisters we discussed above, or close family members.

Keeping things to yourself can also help to keep them low profile. When you share things with a lot of people, no matter if they are close friends, relatives or important to you, your volatility increases unnecessarily. Do recognise that increased importance of those people to us, equals increased exposure to stress loads. There is a happy medium between swallowing it all yourself and spreading it around the whole village. Talking to one or two gatekeepers is the best strategy for everyone concerned.

Reveal no more than necessary

There are people who like to go into minute detail about everything they have done with almost everyone. Sharing things that aren't necessary to or instrumental in achieving your goals may only harm you later on, and revealing every detail keeps you busy learning nothing.

It's in listening and not speaking that we learn. If talking is made of silver, being silent is made of gold. It reveals wisdom, self-discipline and strength of character. Someone who has no secrets is not interesting and attracts a similarly uninspiring crowd, while someone who talks less attracts people who want to discover more about him or her.

Judge situations, not people

If our only interest in conflict is to judge the people involved, then we may end up with few or even no friends at all. On the one hand, we have genetics and neurotransmitter profiles which define our characters and how we respond to stress. On the other, we have the environmental conditions we are in, which impact greatly on shaping us and making us respond in a certain way. To understand a situation deeply, we need to investigate not only what happened and who did it, but also why it happened. What were the circumstances that led someone to act in that way? And we don't want to limit ourselves to only the visible circumstances but also the invisible ones, where the real triggers are often hidden.

MEHDI'S CASE

Mehdi, an IT engineer and father, enjoys living in stressful situations and is a source of stress in his social circle. He is not able to keep his distance from people. Remember the social circle and the solar system? He is either so close to his friends and family members that he becomes a burden on them and ultimately clashes with them, or distances himself, in which case his friends and family lose him for months or even years. He is not able to maintain his orbit.

I wasn't able to help Mehdi directly. All we tried failed – he ended up either leaving or crashing, no matter what. The only thing we could do was to work on his social circle to make them aware of this as much as possible and give them the understanding of the solar system analogy. Once they understood, they are able to deal with him in the right way, contacting him whenever he is drifting away and keep him at a reasonable distance when he is coming dangerously close.

If you know someone like Mehdi and have figured out how to help them, please contact me and share your experience.

13
Mastering Financial Stress

'Money is usually attracted, not pursued.'
— Jim Rohn

Everyone has some sort of financial stress related to their income or how much they own. Wealthy people fear losing what they have, even if fewer material goods could mean less stress.

The more we have, the more our stress triggers multiply. It's a paradox, but that's how people have felt about money since they first created it. Few would be willing to give up part of their wealth in exchange for less stress. On the other hand, low wage earners have noticeably fewer responsibilities, at least in terms of their impact on others, but they have another kind of stress which is more existential in nature.

The only people who are less prone to suffer from this kind of stress are people with a growth mindset. They don't fear losing their jobs or businesses. They might have gone down that road already or feel that they haven't reached their true purpose yet, so they see transition as a challenge to do better and know how to make themselves or their businesses financially successful again.

Let's now have a look at a few techniques to master financial stress by ingraining growth mindset in yourself and making yourself as independent as you can be.

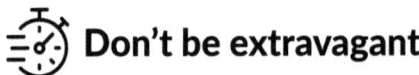 Don't be extravagant

This one is simple: don't buy things you can't afford. If you do so, your dependency on creditors will be like carrying a heavy rock in your rucksack. It will cause your stress levels to multiply all the time until you free yourself by paying your debts off.

Don't buy or invest in anything you don't really need or are not passionate about, even if you can afford it. Happiness bought by money is superficial. True happiness is being self-sufficient with what you have and making minimal investments.

Lead by love and example

There are two main styles of leading if you have responsibility for staff. You can lead by using the power of pressure and fear, or you can lead with the power of love and compassion.

What the first option does is clear. It may give you the impression that you are meeting your targets, but you will dig a deep trench between you and your staff in the twinkling of an eye. In no time, your staff will start to despise you, but because they can't tell you this, it will manifest itself in them hating their work. They will sabotage everything you want to achieve, and sooner or later, they will leave. It's always much easier to destroy reputation, relationships and trust than to build them.

Let your employees love you. Be grateful to them when they do well, help them get better when they fail and encourage them, never blame them. Remember that negative input will be amplified exponentially. A good word can make them happy for a day or two, but a bad word will drag their spirits down for a week or more.

You can also help them outside work. You don't have to change their tyres when they are flat, but just asking about Jane's ill father or John's football training will make their day.

Help employees to do their jobs better by supporting them to learn, develop and grow. It's better that they leave with a high profile than stay on with a low one.

Progress and grow

Learn and progress independently from the business you are in and from your social level. If you stagnate and stop learning and progressing, whether you are working for someone else or for yourself, you'll make yourself redundant and increase the risk of losing your employment if your next boss doesn't like you or your business is outdated. It's like a ticking bomb, which will blow up sooner or later.

As soon as you feel you have learned all aspects of your current job or business and have hit a plateau, focus on developing skills which will enable you to make your current position secure or create new revenue sources for your business. Who stops learning starts to die. Multiplying your skills in areas where you are an absolute specialist in your profession(s) will provide you with a much stronger base to secure your competitiveness and position. The more you know and can put into practice, the safer you will be and the fewer headaches and stresses you will have.

Knowing just one thing is like jumping from a plane with only one parachute. Being able to produce results or solve problems in different areas is like having an enhanced safety net, a second parachute.

Peanuts get monkeys

When it comes to learning, don't be afraid to invest some money to learn first-hand. This is an important technique as most people try to learn on the cheap or through Google and wonder why they haven't moved forward come every birthday.

If you really want to be at the peak of your performance and let employment or projects and investors look for you rather than the other way around, you need to reach deep into your pockets to invest in your education. You can never spend too much on it. Spending to gain access to privileged knowledge will make you unique in your field. It's like buying a few years of lead-time to be ahead of others.

Work on the weak link

Many people focus on their strengths because they feel at home or fear the unknown or change. Be different. Always focus on the weakest links and learn the things you fear or lack as they are the things which will progress you the furthest.

Anticipate a sinking ship

Regardless of whether you are a business owner or an employee, you need to have foresight. When you know the ship is sinking irreversibly, anticipate disaster and sell up or leave before it's too late. On the way out you'll have some cortisol spikes but spare yourself and your time from sinking too. Sell, cut your losses or adapt to change.

Build an independent business

If you run a business that slows down or grinds to a halt when you are on holiday, then you have a big problem. In this case, you have probably always done everything yourself, possibly because you are a perfectionist and don't trust anyone else to perform the required tasks well enough. You may have created a business which works perfectly well when you are around, but as soon as you're away for a day or two, the standards drop and you may have to answer phone calls or emails from your staff every hour or so to give your advice or opinion.

If you have such a business, rethink your strategy. Start by instilling some fundamental changes. Ideally, your business should run by itself, so you can free your time to lean back or grow. You need to hire smartly, delegate tasks and train your staff to be productive and independent. This is a long process so you need to anticipate it early enough to give your employees adequate time to learn to think proactively. But remember that your employees will never feel the same way about your business as you do, even if they are reliable and independent. You have got to keep an eye on things, and they need to know you're doing so.

Build a business you love

If you want to reduce the overall stress load from your business, focus on the word 'love' from beginning to end. This is how to do so:

- Choose a niche in which you feel at home, where working is a pleasure. Doing what you don't like is a stressor. Doing what you love is full of accomplishment.
- Once you've started your dream business, it soaks up your resources. It needs material supplies, hardware assets, finances and employees to survive and grow, until you reach a breakthrough and it becomes profitable. It also needs spiritual and ethical education to help build its mindset and character.
- You have to protect your business from external harm. Working with clients you don't feel comfortable with will stress you. Choose your clients wisely – you want the ones with the same type of work ethic as yours – and don't allow

yourself to accept all kinds. This will make you happy and fill your business with joy. Don't waste your energy working with difficult clients; this will drain you and suck out your energy. Sense who the potential problem clients are and tell them – in a friendly way – to get lost.

Passive and active staff

Staff will never feel the same way about a business as the owner does. They simply can't. Only the owner will know the numbers and be sensitive in regard to the survival and growth of the business, but this doesn't mean there isn't room for optimisation.

You may on the one hand have a minority of staff who think proactively and want to grow, but there's always the risk they will start their own business if they get the chance. On the other hand, you may have passive staff who are happy doing the bare minimum and don't like to be under the spotlight. The right hiring and staff training techniques are crucial for getting loyal staff who want to grow with the company. Make sure to create an atmosphere of motivation and equality with opportunities for growth and progress.

Nothing costs a company more than having trained staff leaving suddenly. Candidates who are always looking for jobs with higher salaries will leave the company at the drop of a hat and will be unlikely to address problems with the boss. They will just make their decision, announce it and leave. Be attentive, read the signs carefully and be ready for all eventualities.

Price doesn't always equal value

Some people fall into the high-price, high-value trap, especially in today's world where the market is overfilled with things everyone is supposed to need and a product comes in multiple versions with a broad price range. Surely it must be good if it is expensive?

Price can correlate to quality as it will give the producers the finances they need to improve their products, but it's not always the case. If we focus on price alone and always opt for the most expensive options without even looking at all possibilities, then we are wasting big money which could be invested in other projects. This is especially painful for someone on a tight budget as it creates a load of financial stress. Price is not the only criterion for good quality; it's better to study all the details and reviews of a product or service prior to buying it. It might be that goods with a lower price will be of better quality and durability.

Define your required value of a thing prior to purchase

Even if the quality of a product or service is worth the money, sometimes we don't need the highest level of quality. We need to ask ourselves how we will use that item, how often and for how long.

When I worked designing nuclear power plants, I used different classifications to express different requirements for a part, piece of equipment, sensor, valve, piping line, electrical cable or door. Every item, from the smallest to the biggest, was classified depending on its required functionality and availability. If my colleagues and I had chosen the highest classification of all parts, then a power station would have cost many times more with no added benefit.

We all have the potential in our daily lives to save resources by focusing on our real requirements of the things we buy rather than going for the best every time. They should be able to provide those requirements and no more. Our first step is to define the requirements, then look for the right item to cover them.

The savings and financial freedom when you apply this technique in the long run are too huge to be ignored. Maybe those savings could help you change profession, learn something new or create more independence one day.

Your ability to make money is more important than money

Of course, having a certain amount of money in your bank account or tied up in valuable goods or property reduces stress linked to finances as it gives you some security should something go wrong one day. But more important than money itself is the ability to make it. This gives you far more freedom and peace of mind.

When a skilled martial artist or boxer has learned the finer techniques of self-defence, he or she will not be stressed about walking down the darkest of roads at night as they'll know they have the ability to defend themselves and others. Some people take it as a personal challenge to start from scratch to make big money, but their main asset is their brain. They have acquired the right skills to become a genius in creativity and organisation while maintaining an enduring and cool mind. No one is born with these skills just as no one is born able to perform martial arts, but once someone has gone through experience and exposure, nothing can shock them anymore.

I'm not suggesting you give away everything you have and learn to earn it all back again from scratch. The moral of this technique is to be cautious and learn the skills from others who have been through hardships. Learn from their mistakes and successes.

Don't be your own worst enemy by not believing in your capabilities. Maybe you can do better than a lot of people out there who have gained experience and succeeded. Sharpen your axe and be prepared for the eventuality that you may lose everything; don't just be scared and stressed about how much you have to lose.

SELMA'S CASE

Selma loved spending money. On top of that, she would always look for the most expensive options when she was buying things. She wouldn't even consider looking for cheaper alternatives, and this applied to all kinds of purchases, from tissues to cars and even houses.

Her excessive spending and opting for the most expensive options put her whole family into high levels of stress, especially when she borrowed money to buy things she couldn't afford. She always armed herself with a load of arguments to defend her point of view until she had bought what she desired. Sometimes when she knew her arguments weren't strong enough, she'd buy what she wanted in secret, then the delivery arrived and everyone was faced with the bitter truth.

Unfortunately, after only a few days of enjoying a new purchase, Selma would become bored with it and her instinct would kick in again for a new adventure. This led to her children avoiding her when she tried to get them on her side to win an argument with her husband, and her husband feeling under pressure at all times.

Looking back to when she was young, Selma realised she was always a rebel who had never accepted her parents' decisions, even though they were very strict with her. The combination of being a rebel and coming from a poor family led to her extreme way of spending money.

The highest stress test for the whole family was when she decided to buy a house. Of course, she wanted the biggest one with the largest garden in the village. She opted for a house the family couldn't afford and clearly she and her husband couldn't ever pay back the mortgage in their lifetime.

After months of fights and negotiations with her husband, she won and they signed the construction contract. She and her family were trapped with a tight budget, and her extravagant choices to fit out the house with top-of-the-range options didn't help. The stress was so high that she started feeling sick and weak.

It was obvious when she came to me for help that it wouldn't make a lot of sense to argue with her to convince her to change her habit. What I asked put her in a position of deep self-reflection. I asked her whether the person who she was working for as a cleaner would be able to afford the kind of house she was planning to buy. She took few moments to think about it, and then admitted that her own employer wouldn't be able to afford even a cheaper house.

I'm not sure if it was my question that led to it, but now Selma has completely changed. She is not buying new things; instead, her husband buys what she really needs for her and she has learned to enjoy what she has for a longer period of time. She can now save money for a better education for her kids.

14
Managing Environmental Stress

'Humans are the only species bright enough to make artificial light and stupid enough to live under it.'
— Jack Kruse

This type of stress is triggered by our immediate surroundings. It could be the environment we work in, live in, or if we choose to be predominantly outside in nature or indoors. Some of its stress triggers can only be reduced, but never totally removed. Changing our environment needs a big plan, commitment, decisive power and willingness.

Let's have a look at some practical solutions we can apply to reduce this type of stress.

Information abstention

If you are consuming information you don't need which is causing unnecessary stress, you can choose to block it. For example, if you're sitting in a cab and watching all the cars on the street or looking at advertisements or listening to negative news on the driver's radio, the amount the information you're absorbing is relatively high, but you could block it out by reading something or just closing your eyes and listening to a podcast. You then abstain from consuming unnecessary information to reduce your stress load.

Mind unnecessary sounds

Unnatural sounds, such as those made by a train, car or machine, or background noises like those produced by a PC or air conditioner often stress us more than natural ones. In contrast, the sound of waves, rain or a plunging waterfall calms us down. Even violent natural noises like roaring thunder, a raging storm or a rumbling volcano, although they may scare the heck out of us, still make us listen with wonder.

Unnatural noises don't just stress us, they can lower our IQ. An interesting study done prior and after the relocation of the airport of Munich has shown that prior to the relocation high noise exposure was associated with deficits in long-term memory and reading comprehension. Two years after the airport closure those deficits disappeared. The same deficits were found in children living in the vicinity of the new airport.[106]

Protect your ears whenever you can to lower the noise coming from the emitters around you. At the same time, ignore or block the reception of the noises you can't switch off. If you are working in a multi-boxed office and there are peaks of sound levels coming from your colleagues or other devices, plug in earplugs to avoid stress loads and help you concentrate on performing your tasks better. I would advise you to use earplugs whenever you encounter stressful noise levels and you can't reduce them. Typical examples are on a plane, on a busy road (as long as you're not driving) or while operating heavy machinery.

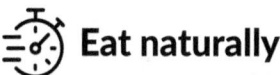

Eat naturally

Every time we return to nature, it has a positive impact on our stress response, and food is no exception. Eating processed foods has the opposite effect. It leaves us inflamed and bloated, and the resultant surge of empty calories will cause our mood and energy to crash before long. All of this will stress us.

Sugary food and artificial ingredients are designed to make us addicted so we continue buying and

---

[106] Monika Bullinger et al., 'The psychological cost of aircraft noise for children' (2012), https://doi.org/10.1016/S0934-8859(99)80014-5

consuming more of the same. Natural food, as expensive as it may be, is vastly superior to processed food. In terms of the quality of food and supplements, don't compare on the basis of price, especially where bad-quality foods are concerned. Rather, compare food on the basis of health benefits. How precious is the health of your immune system, liver, heart and brain to you? When you consider this, every penny you're paying for bad-quality food, you're actually (and foolishly) spending on buying disease and inflammation. Natural food grows on trees or comes from the ground, the sea or the sky. If it doesn't, then you can be 100% sure it's aggressive and inflammatory.

Eating natural foods makes us one with nature and refuels us with a balanced mix of macro and micronutrients. This ultimately leaves us with happy cortisol levels.

Extreme temperatures

Being exposed to cold after increasing our body temperature through exercising or being in the sauna has a huge impact on the endorphins and hormones we release. Cold temperatures impact our testosterone levels and kick start our immune system. Hot temperatures impact our GH levels, especially if we're exposed to them right after our strength training session.

Expose your body to a wide range of temperatures. Don't overheat your space during winter and don't overcool it in the summer. Use saunas and cold showers or ice baths. You can start by submerging your face in ice-cold water in a sink at home and progress from there.

Don't fear complexity

Never be afraid of objects and subjects that appear complex. If something seems complex, it tends to be primarily because the person who is presenting it hasn't yet found an easy way to do it. Every subject is just an accumulation of interrelated information, so it's possible to break anything down into bits of information as simple as true or false, one or zero (which is how all computers and smart devices work).

If you are faced with a task which seems to be complex, remember this and break it down. Digest every piece independently. You will finish by unravelling the complexity, leading to clarity and understanding. Look for the best explanation. It also helps to keep this in mind so you can explain things clearly to others.

Usually, the more complex things seem to be, the more time and the smaller the steps we need to break them down. If we have a complex maths demonstration to give, for example, focusing on the start and the end will confuse us and diffuse our energy. We need to break the whole demonstration into small steps and understand each one independently. Once we've understood, we can move on to the next until we get to the final result.

Your space

Your home and office have something in common: you spend most of your time in one or the other, so you want to implement corrective actions such as lowering your exposure to EMF, artificial light, grounding etc. Do this in those two places first, and progress from there.

Set everything up to make it as comfortable and motivating as possible so you can be productive and achieve your peak performance. Nothing should be disturbing or missing. Promote productivity on one hand and recovery and recharging on the other.

Why not have an espresso machine or water boiler next to your desk in your office, or an infrared sauna at home? Be your own king or queen and reward yourself accordingly if you are working for peak performance. Make sure you have everything you need to work hard and be a peak achiever, and also have everything you need to recover well.

Go back to nature

I'm sure you don't need a book like this to realise that living in lush surroundings is far more beneficial to your health and stress management than living in cities. Ashes to ashes, dust to dust – our body comes from the earth, grows with nature (which is one of the reasons why processed food is so bad for us, by the way) and is recycled back into the earth. People who have lost or cut their connection to nature live an unnatural life. If you don't believe me, compare city folk to farmers; someone who has grown up in a concrete jungle against someone who has grown his or her own vegetables and fruit.

If you live in a city, regularly go out into nature, for example have a trip into the countryside every weekend. If you have family who live in the country, visit them often, and if they are farmers, help them work on the land. Get involved, get dirty and work with animals. Inhale fresh air and eat fresh food.

You could also look towards moving out of the city. Remember this when you are looking for a new job or moving to a new place.

Be rough

All the devices, gadgets and tools we have to make our lives more comfortable and make us better at what we do are instead making us weak and dependent on them. When we are weak, a general state of unhappiness prevails in our life, which is typically followed sooner or later by depression and anxiety.

Why take the car if we can walk? Why take the lift if we can climb the stairs? Why use the navigation system if we can use our sense of orientation? Why use the calculator if we can do the maths in our brains? Why use artificial lighting if we can use sunlight or candlelight? Why use air conditioning if our body is designed to adapt to extreme temperatures? And the list goes on.

Cars and lifts are making us fatter and lazier. Navigation systems make us lose our sense of orientation. The calculator makes us under-stimulate our brain, which may respond by regressing. Electronic screens and artificial lighting are destroying our circadian rhythm and causing havoc in our body. Air conditioning makes our body forget about its capacity to adapt to a wide range of temperatures and humidity, which has a profound impact on our motivation and determination. When was the last time you took an ice-cold shower? Do you remember how you felt just after?

Reducing gadgets to the absolute minimum brings us closer to nature and makes us independent and strong. Feeling this rough strength calms us, reduces our anxiety and increases our happiness. Note, this isn't contradicting the 'Your space' technique. You can use all the tools necessary to help you achieve your peak performance and recovery, but still be minimalist in your tools of choice. There is a happy medium which you'll need to identify for yourself.

Smart use of smart devices

We live in times where the majority of people believe they are not able to function properly if they are not online. Being online has become as essential as being able to breathe. There are relatively few people who realise how stressful it is to be online all the time and take steps to reduce their toxic electro-exposure.

Train yourself to live without smartphones and other smart devices. Define a certain time where your smartphone is switched off and remains untouched. Start with a short time window on weekends and progress from there. Find more useful replacement activities to fill the time you have freed, like reading a book or learning a beneficial skill such as cooking.

Never play a game on your smartphone. Even if you have got some time to kill, playing on smart devices activates the frontal part of the brain by releasing dopamine, which in turn makes you more addicted to it. Apply the 'as low as reasonably applicable' (ALARA) principle to electronic devices. Be smart; get that thing under control before it gets you under control.

Junk light

All artificial lighting, smart devices and electronic displays are emitters of an unnatural wave spectrum. They primarily emit blue light, which is not harmful in itself if it's coming from a natural source like the sun or fire as it is then balanced by infrared light. But coming from artificial light and electronic displays, it is disruptive to our circadian rhythm and mitochondrial functions.

When the retina senses blue light, it has an adverse impact on melatonin production and gives false information to our brains that the day has just started. The body replies by secreting cortisol to supply more glucose into the bloodstream as it believes it needs energy, which is not true under such circumstances. We end up with heightened cortisol, glucose and insulin levels late in the evening when we actually want all of those three to be at their minimum.

Sensed blue light at the cellular level interferes with the mitochondrial processes of energy production. This will lower the mitochondrial activity of our cells, in turn lowering our energy reserves in general.

A study has shown that artificial light induces ACTH production, the role of which is to trigger cortisol secretion by the adrenals, by the hypothalamus. Prof Dr Hollwich, who conducted this research, says:

'Increasing the intensity of artificial light with "neon-tubes" (fluorescent tubes) leads to "light stress" proved by increased hormone production – especially the stress hormone cortisol. The belief that artificial light is the same as natural light, and that it can fully replace it, is inappropriate in the medical view and needs correction'.[107]

This is how you can apply the ALARA principle here:

- Protect your eyes by wearing protective blue-light-blocking glasses when you are indoors or using electronic displays.

- Adjust the light of your displays to a more natural tone. Usually, you can do this by putting it on nightshift mode, thereby reducing the blue-light peak.

- Cover your skin to protect your mitochondria from being exposed to blue light.

- Expose your skin to direct sunlight, especially in the mornings, to establish more balance and mitigate the harmful effects of artificial lighting.

Blue light sensed by the retina and the skin relays information to the mitochondria to produce more free

---

[107] F Hollwich and B Dieckhues, 'Der Einfluss des Lichtes über das Auge auf den Stoffwechsel und die Hormone' [author's own translation from German: 'Effect of light on the eye on metabolism and hormones] (1989), www.ncbi.nlm.nih.gov/pubmed/2557485

radicals.[108] Red light gives the opposite information to the mitochondria, stopping the free radical production and cleaning them up. Knowing that mitochondria are overproducing free radicals, the cells dissolve them. We end up having less mitochondria, which means less energy.

Mind toxins

Toxicity is all around us. We even buy it in our skincare products or, worse still, food. Unfortunately, we can only talk about minimising its effects and being best placed to deal with it.

Here, information is key. If we don't know the sources of toxicity, its effects and how we can keep them at bay, then we are taking a huge risk at the expense of our health. The strategy against toxicity is to reduce exposure on the one hand and strengthen ourselves through supplying the macro and micronutrients needed during the detoxification processes on the other. We can also perform regular detox mitigation such as IR Sauna, soft tissue treatment or supplemental detox.

Toxicity is an additional stress load on our bodies because it can alter our physiological processes. It

---

108 B F Godley, 'Blue light induces mitochondrial DNA damage and free radical production in epithelial cells' (2005), www.ncbi.nlm.nih.gov/pubmed/15797866

MANAGING ENVIRONMENTAL STRESS

can even mimic hormones and trigger corresponding signals. Xeno-oestrogens are toxins that can mimic oestrogens and trigger the response cascade such as storing fat, in men as well as women. Bisphenol A (BPA), which is contained in many food-packaging products, is able to disrupt the whole endocrine system and can double our risk of becoming diabetic if a concentration of more than 5 µg/L is found in our urine.[109]

The majority of toxins are unnatural molecules, like vapour or exhaust fumes from petrochemicals and chemical products used in food or plastics. These molecules find their way into our system by being inhaled, as is the case with exhaust fumes, pesticides and insecticides being ingested with food or water, or coming into contact with our skin via skincare or haircare products etc. In extreme cases, they can be implanted into us in dental fillings, or silicone or plastic implants through cosmetic surgery.

Once toxins get into the bloodstream, they get into the liver, which will then try to get rid of them by detoxification processes. There are different phases of detoxification which need raw materials to finish the physiological reaction. If we have poor eating habits, the detoxification process cannot finish, and sometimes it can't even start. The toxins remain in the

---

[109] J Pizzorno, *The Toxin Solution: How hidden poisons in the air, water, food and products we use are destroying our health and what we can do to fix it* (HarperCollins, 2007).

bloodstream until they are stored in fat cells, including in the brain in cases of heavy metals like cadmium, arsenic and lead.

Here are some techniques that are specific to protecting ourselves from the source of toxins.

In air (gaseous or solid particles):

- Primarily, choose where you live. Living in the country is always best, but you need to make sure the area is low in toxins and doesn't have polluters like a coal-fired power plant or petrochemical or pharmaceutical plant in the vicinity.
- Avoid driving a diesel car and try not to inhale vaporised and evaporating gases when refuelling your car.
- Ventilate your car when you get in, especially on sunny days. Wind down all the windows and turn the aeration system to maximum flow to replace the car's interior atmosphere with fresh air. Sun heats up your car interior, which then releases nasty chemicals from all the plastic fixtures and surfaces.
- Monitor air toxicity and, if needed, use a gas mask or stay at home.

In food (liquid or solid):

- Ban and boycott food containing pesticides and chemicals
- Don't use plastic to store or consume your food or beverages
- Don't use pans with stick-free film or non-stick coatings
- Always boil your water in stainless steel and never in plastic boilers

In skincare (liquid or gaseous):

- Use natural cosmetic products
- Use natural cleaning products for laundry and the kitchen
- Use a water filter in your shower if needed

You can refer to the Environmental Working Group for more information about the products you can safely use.[110]

Detoxify

In terms of strengthening our body, we need to know that our main detoxification organs besides the liver

---

110 www.ewg.org

are our gut and kidneys. The liver filters the toxins out from the blood and then launches the detoxification process, which transforms the toxin into molecules that are easily excreted. There are different detoxification phases,[111] all of which need different macro or micronutrients such as vitamins, amino acids etc to occur successfully. Toxins ingested with food or water are absorbed into the bloodstreams in the gut, hence the importance of an intact gut lining and a nutrition high in fibre to reduce the toxic influx. The kidneys are important to excrete the toxins via the urinary pathway.

To provide the raw materials for the detoxification process, a good starting strategy would be to combine a diet which is nutrient-rich, including a variety of protein sources, colourful vegetables, fibres and antioxidants, together with complementary supplementation. Our nutrition alone will never be able to cover all our needs, due to the poor quality of our food on the one hand and the increased influx of toxins on the other, so we need to complement our nutrition with the right amount of high-grade supplementation, such as essential anti-inflammatory fats and minerals.

Secondly, the right frequency of meals is essential. Usually a fasting period is good for detoxification, but if fasting is not for you, then eat meals every 2.5 to 3

---

111 The conventional medical school speaks about two phases, the functional approach speaks about three and more phases. We will address this in detail in the second pillar: *Eat Better, Feel Greater*.

hours to supply important nutrients to the liver on a regular basis.

Last but not least, drinking enough water is key to help the body dilute and flush toxins out from the organs. There is a lot of research about the optimal amount, which depends on gender, activity level, body weight, time of the year and location etc, but as a rule of thumb, drinking around 3.7 L per day for adults is a safe level to aim for. Think about timing your intake and reduce it gradually in the late afternoon to ensure you don't interrupt your sleep.

You can also consider regular detox sessions in your overall strategy to eliminate toxins. The more toxins your environment has, the more often you'll need to detoxify.

You could implement one or a combination of:

- Regular IR sauna
- Regular soft tissue treatment such as the Chinese Gua Sha to help mobilise toxins
- High-fibre cure to fix toxins and help with their excretion
- Specific supplemental detox cure for heavy metals
- Regular strength training

Bear in mind that you have to take care of your main detoxification organs – gut, liver and kidneys – and inform your doctor prior to starting on a detoxification programme.

Beware of mould

Depending on the humidity level, temperature, architecture and heating, ventilation and air conditioning of the buildings we spend our time in, we may have unwanted 'guests' living with us. Everyone has probably seen the dark green or black layer on the silicone sealing around the bathroom sink or bathtub, on ceilings when rooms are not properly ventilated or in water-damaged buildings.

Not all types of mould are toxic, but there are some nasty ones, and some people may be highly sensitive to these. Certain types of mould generate biotoxins to survive, and these can have a disastrous impact on us. Upon intruding into our bloodstreams, these biotoxins are able to switch off our immune system and dock on to cell receptor sites, which then create havoc in our body by activating autoimmune genes. Once those genes are turned on, the inflammation process goes violently out of control.[112]

---

112 P Schmidt, *Mold Warriors: Fighting America's hidden health threat* (Gateway Press, 2005).

With an altered immune system, toxins generate all kinds of nasty conditions including multiple sclerosis, blood clotting, obesity, chronic fatigue and cancer. The body fights to move toxins from the liver to the upper intestines, but the toxins get reabsorbed prior to being excreted and so we enter into an endless cycle.

Living with mould may lead to an overproduction of cytokines, which are able to bind and lock the receptor sites used by leptin at the hypothalamus. The result is an overproduction of leptin, which leads to leptin resistance. Leptin resistance leads our body to be efficient at storing fat and being unable to lose it, feeling more tired and being in pain. A leptin resistant person stores fat much easier than a leptin sensitive person, even if both are on the same caloric surplus. Stubborn fat storage, being highly sensitive to pain and chronic fatigue are all harbingers of catastrophic conditions.

Mould and its effects are a detailed topic beyond the scope of this book, but we do need take mould seriously. If we fail to do so, we may nullify all our efforts to live a healthy life or lose fat by putting ourselves on a hamster wheel. I strongly advise you to study the work of Dr R Shoemaker, who is the pioneer in this field.[113]

---

113 www.survivingmold.com

STEPHAN'S CASE

I had the pleasure of working with Stephan, a German safety engineer, on a 12-week health transformation. After fixing his sleep, adjusting his nutrition and starting with efficient strength training in the second week, he saw his body fat starting to melt away.

The laws of physiology and metabolism apply to everybody, but they may apply differently. One client may start losing fat right away, another one might be resistant at the beginning. In Stephan's case, he saw big fat losses quickly to start with, but he stagnated at about midway. His abdominal skin fold stayed in place for a few weeks, despite him sticking to the demanding workouts and doing everything else as per the programme.

I looked at his diet, then any environmental stressors such as smartphone antennas or smart meters etc, but I couldn't find anything which could be the reason for his stagnation. But when he invited me to his home, I was shocked to discover that the corners of the rooms and a few areas on the ceilings in his bathroom and kitchen were covered with the black spots of mould and I quickly made the link to his stagnation. I suggested he detoxify his home, and then go through a detox programme himself, which he did. Still we couldn't see any progress in the weeks after.

While he was away on a business trip, he sent me some pictures and I could see that his lower abdomen was getting smaller. When he next came in and we measured his skin folds, we discovered they were way below where they had been when he plateaued and the fat on his lower abdomen had almost disappeared, indicating that the toxic load from the mould was without doubt responsible for his stagnation.

Now we have covered managing environmental stress, it's time to move on to the final type of stress: nutritional.

15
Mastering Nutritional Stress

'Depression is an inflammatory disease.'
— Dr David Perlmutter

Bizarrely, despite our massive advancements in technology, our food quality has gone down dramatically. Genetically modified foods, pro-inflammatory foods and those loaded with chemicals like pesticides have become the norm for the masses. While our ancestors ate 100% biological food, this has become a rare exception for us.

Poor dietary choices result in increased oxidative stress. Let's take the example of trans fats, which are widely used in the food industry. Trans fats are highly pro-inflammatory as they attack every cell, including brain cells, and may cause cognitive decline.[114] Refined sugars or carbohydrates in general combined with bad insulin sensitivity oxidise cholesterol, which is then blamed for heart diseases and high blood pressure.

Another example is gluten. According to a number of studies there is a clear link between gluten sensitivity and neurological disorders. It's not just relevant for people with the celiac disease but for almost every one of us. Dr Perlmutter mentions in his work that 40 percent of us can't properly process gluten and the remaining 60 percent could be in harm's way.[115] A great number of people have issues with gluten but don't realise it. Only at a later stage, with early signs of dementia and Alzheimer's disease, do we feel the effects which gluten has on our cognitive function.

All of these examples stress the body and its vital organs. Pro-inflammatory foods trigger inflammations in the gut. A continuous state of inflammation will sooner or later produce big holes in the gut lining, known as permeation. These holes would allow longer molecules, which have not been completely digested yet, and bacteria to enter the bloodstream, keeping the immune system working overtime to fight an endless war. The results are overall inflammation of the body and its organs, including the brain,

---

114 N D Barnard, A E Bunner and U Agarwal, 'Saturated and trans fats and dementia: a systematic review' (2014), www.ncbi.nlm.nih.gov/pubmed/24916582
115 D Perlmutter, *The Grain Brain* (Hodder & Stoughton, 2018).

weak immune system, low energy, mood swings and depression.

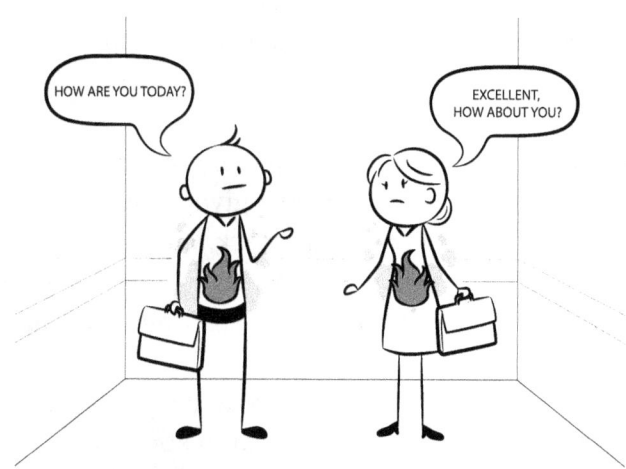

An interesting study has shown that what we eat and drink will impact our epigenome, which is our genetic material.[116] This study shows the importance of 'saint' food not only for ourselves, but also for generations to come as our epigenome may be inherited.

A second kind of nutritional stress is due to our consumption of coffee, tea and other stimulants. They're not bad per se, but we need to notice that they raise cortisol as a response and give consideration to when we consume them.

A third kind of nutritional stress is related to when we're eating or not eating. A nutritional regime with

---

[116] MJ Dauncey, 'Recent advances in nutrition, genes and brain health' (2012), www.ncbi.nlm.nih.gov/pubmed/22716958/

feeding windows that are too large or a low frequency of meals, as many of us follow, or fasting can lead to an increase in cortisol levels. I'm not saying that fasting is a bad thing as I believe it has its benefits, but we have to realise that not eating has this result.

The last kind of nutritional stress is when we set up a nutritional regime to achieve a given goal, but don't commit to it and keep falling back to old eating habits. For some people, this is like being on the hamster wheel and it produces peak stresses when they fail.

Let's discuss a few techniques to allow you to reduce nutritional stress by getting inflammation under control and establishing a good gut flora, which is great for the body and brain.

Gut rebuilding

If you have been consuming food which has led to gut inflammation and leaky gut, consult with your doctor or nutritionist and ask for help to establish a healthy gut flora. The strategy could be to deal with the inflammation by identifying and eliminating the problematic food and stopping its consumption, and using supplements like essential fatty acids and curcumin. The next step would be to seal your gut lining with regular glutamine intake, which is an amino acid and is the building block of the junction cells. The last step would be to use probiotics to introduce good bacteria.

You need more fat than sugar

Many of us have been criticising a real friend for far too long, and we are still doing it. I often have discussions with clients and friends who think fat is bad and leads to cardiovascular issues and obesity. Once a bad impression has been spread in society, it takes ages for science and ambassadors to reverse the perception. It's like when the captain of a big ship changes course, but the inertia of the ship means it needs half an hour to respond. At the same time, we are neglecting the negative effects of the real enemy, which is sugar (especially in a combination of toxins as we have seen above).

Fats are essential; sugars aren't. Fats lubricate our arteries and cells and keep them alive and active; sugars raise the oxidative stress. Fats provide sustainable energy without spiking blood sugar and insulin; sugars inflame the body, gut and brain and leave us with chronically high cortisol levels.

Come back to fat. It's sugar which makes us fat. Embrace a diet with low carbs, high natural fat and high protein, and get lean, fight inflammation and save your brain from sugar.

I'm not against sugars in berries, dates, figs etc, but we have been consuming sugars for so long, we first have to stop them completely for a while to increase our insulin sensitivity. We'll then really deserve them again once we are lean.

Watch your meal frequency

Eating meals too infrequently will increase our cortisol levels as we go hypoglycemic in between them. For example, if we have one small breakfast, and then two bigger meals at lunchtime and dinnertime, we will spike our insulin with each meal. We often love foods with a high glycemic index. This leads to satisfaction as serotonin levels increase, but this is just for a short time as our sinking insulin levels post-spike will make sure that we feel low. Then cortisol levels increase to support a release of energy to the body.

A much better strategy would be to have smaller meals more frequently, fuelled by fat rather than carbohydrates, to stabilise your insulin levels and provide sustained, continuous energy. I'm thinking about meals every 2.5 to 3 hours. A good indicator is when you feel mildly hungry, think about consuming your next meal, but avoid snacking in between. Besides often being loaded with nasty calorific additives, snacks won't help much to stabilise your insulin and sugar levels.

 ## Eat only when the sun is out

A good technique to avoid going to bed with a full stomach is only to eat during the hours of natural daylight. Look to have a 3 to 4 hour window between your last meal and bedtime.

Your morning friend becomes your evening enemy

Natural stimulants like coffee and tea are excellent sources of antioxidants with their neuroprotective properties. This is especially true in the morning, but avoid consuming them too late and too often. You don't want your stimulant consumption to interfere with your circadian rhythm. And if you are running on coffee, you are driving your adrenals nuts.

Your body needs up to 6 hours to excrete the stimulating agent. Add a 2-hour margin and consume your last coffee or black or green tea 8 hours in total before going to bed.

Divorce from allergens

The first step here is to identify the common allergens we are consuming on a regular basis and ban them from our table. Aggressive foods which create havoc in our body are those containing gluten and trans fats. If you are among those who like scientific evidence, then I recommend reading the works of Dr David Perlmutter.[117]

Next, if you still get a bloated belly or any indications of an allergic reaction, eliminate nuts, milk products

---

117 D Perlmutter, *The Grain Brain* (Hodder & Stoughton, 2018).

and grains individually. More often than not, at least one of these triggers allergic reactions.

An easy technique for testing your reactivity to food, which I learned from my mentor Charles R Poliquin, is refeeding after abstention. Abstain from the suspicious food for a few weeks, then on one day eat as much of it as you can and note your reaction. If you feel splendid, then the test has failed and the food is not a trigger for you, but should you feel horrible, then you know to cut that food from your diet.

Take care of your friends

I'm not talking about human friends here, but your gut bacteria. If they are kept in balance, they are working for you and doing a wonderful job. They help you digest food, release neurotransmitters and develop a strong immune system.[118] If you feed them well by supplying enough fibres, good fats and proteins with moderate complex carb consumption, then you establish a balanced gut flora. In this case, your immune system will be healthy and your body free from inflammation and oxidative stress.

If you consume more starchy and glutinous carbs, pro-inflammatory fats and processed meats, then you'll establish an imbalanced gut flora, a condition which

---

118 V Robles Alonso and F Guarner, 'Linking the gut microbiota to human health' (2013), www.ncbi.nlm.nih.gov/pubmed/23360877

is also called dysbiosis. In this case, your gut becomes inflamed which results in permeability, allowing long and undigested food molecules and bacteria into the bloodstream. Once this happens, your immune system will never rest again and the inflammation will be spread all over your body, even knocking at your brain's door. That's real stress for your entire system.

What you like may not like you

Remember that you need variety in your nutrition. Eating something too often will lead to reactions and cross-reactions. Forget about bodybuilders who claim to eat chicken at all times. Invest time in learning to cook a variety of foods and reward yourself with good health. Your body is worth it.

Clean up your kitchen

If you are on a specific diet such as gluten free, ketogenic or low carb, then clean all sources of your banned substances from your kitchen. If you don't have them in your home, you are less likely to fall back on them. Put yourself in a much better place to succeed and reduce the related stress to the minimum.

If you can't do that, then avoid being in the kitchen late in the evening as this is when you are more likely to crave sugar to produce more serotonin. This is also another good reason to go to bed early.

Fasting

Fasting has many important benefits which makes it interesting to consider. Imagine a life without fasting. Your digestive system would be working nonstop and your night's sleep would be too short to give it a meaningful break.

Besides detoxification, promoting insulin sensitivity and having a positive impact on fighting cancer cell development, fasting all day long teaches us patience, which is a good quality for mastering stress. But we still need to remember that physiologically, fasting raises our cortisol levels, so it might not be the best option to fast when we have chronically high cortisol levels or adrenal insufficiency. We should first master our stress and cortisol levels, only then consider fasting.

Lifestyle versus dieting

If you force yourself on to a diet which is too restrictive without the right frequency of mealtimes and reward, you may end up going nuts and eating every sweet you can find. This is known as binging. Depending on your carbohydrate tolerance, you may be able to handle a carb meal once in a while. There are people who can eat rice nonstop without getting fat and there are others who can barely handle the smell. This all depends on your genetic makeup and how your ancestors used to feed themselves.

If you don't tolerate carbs well and you cut them too drastically, you may become their slave. Often, serotonin-driven people, when out of balance, binge on carbs to replace their low serotonin levels. It's natural but damaging behaviour. As serotonin concentration increases towards the evening to help with the preparation for sleep and relaxation, often serotonin-driven people start craving sugar and carbs at that time of day.

MARCO'S CASE

When I started coaching Marco, he was in the middle of an extremely stressful phase which he had been enduring for more than 2.5 years. As a super specialist, he had a stressful job with a lot of interactions and responsibilities; he was working for more than 10 hours per day, 6 days a week quite regularly and was over-consuming carbs while doing almost no physical activity.

Adding strength training would only have stressed him even more, so we started by implementing changes in his recovery strategy with the main goal being to increase his sleep length and quality and reduce his stress load so he could start working out. His individualised supplementation programme helped him shift his sleep to normal hours and establish a neurotransmitter balance, and by changing his office, he reduced his workload dramatically. Being a dopamine-driven person, he responded well to what I call a traffic-light diet – zero to low carbs, medium fat, high protein – which boosted his energy levels and made him excel in the gym. He has now not only regained his full brainpower and energy levels, his progress in the gym starting from day one has been phenomenal. I remember his first day in the gym. Marco was not able to perform even one chin up with full range of motion. When he had to move back to his native country he was able to perform just four chin ups with perfect form while gaining 10 kg more on the scale of lean muscle mass and with an additional 27.5 kg attached to his waist.

Conclusion

In this book we have addressed how you can master your sleep and your stress, including the first approach to managing stress, the emitter/receptor approach. Understanding this provides you with an antidote to your personal storms.

Once you include the right techniques for you as part of your lifestyle, your sleep will be reenergising and refuelling. Even if you have nagging concerns caused by priorities and outstanding tasks, jetlag or something you can't avoid, you know exactly what to do to regulate the ill-effects and get back on track. Your stress tolerance will be high and your stress input will always be kept low – this is what this book can help you attain. You'll know what and where all your stress sources are and prioritise placing yourself in the strongest position to manage them. Typically, you'll be thirsty for knowledge and hungry for success. You'll read a lot, always looking for ways to develop yourself, progress and grow. You'll dedicate time, effort and finances to giving back. You'll help anyone in need without expecting anything in return and won't rely on anyone but yourself. This is a kind and altruistic approach to meeting the daily challenges in life.

You now know how to nourish yourself, be healthy and avoid allergens. You can treat each problem as a project to accomplish and learn from the past to have a better future. Your mistakes are chances for improvement and progress rather than failures that need punishing. Each failure makes you more powerful. You can become your strongest critic and have no problem whatsoever with changing your mind when you recognise you've made a mistake or others are in the right.

Look for your gatekeepers and nurture your relationships with them. Love giving more than receiving, transforming selfishness to graciousness. These are the winning ways of successful people, peak achievers and the ones who want to become aces.

Much of what we have covered embraces age-old and time-tested methods to become a more conscious, conscientious, healthy, pleasant and productive person.

CONCLUSION

Scientific research and greater knowledge reflect in today's facilities and lifestyles – all of which we've touched on in this book. You now have the weapons you need to neutralise the downsides of modern living.

Acknowledgements

Thank you to all mentors, brothers and sisters who helped in this work. Special thank you to Debs Jenkins for her great guidance and my brother Alastair Black from www.languageandmore.de for the meticulous proofreading.

The Author

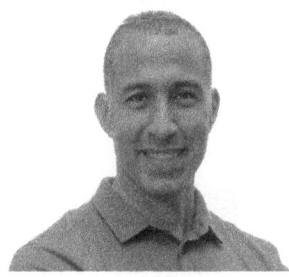

Riad Hechame is a chemical engineer, strength coach, soft tissue practitioner and functional medicine student. His calling, passion and ultimate goal is to lead people to achieve their personal peak human performance by optimising all available and necessary health parameters.

Riad was privileged enough to complete the comprehensive educational curriculum as a student of world-renowned strength coach extraordinaire, Charles R Poliquin. He regularly consults with top experts, researchers and trainers worldwide to remain among the leading players in the strength and performance game. The wealth of knowledge he has harnessed from various mentors blesses him with unique abilities to guide and help high-achievers, both executives and athletes, as well as the general population to realise their potential and achieve ultimate performance.

You can contact Riad at:
Me@RiadHechame.com

Listen to his podcast on iTunes and Stitcher:
Peak Human Performance

Keep up to date with the latest findings and advice on Peak Human Performance at:
www.RiadHechame.com

Take the sleep test at:
www.phpstrengthclinic.com/sleep

Take the stress test at:
www.phpstrengthclinic.com/stress

www.ingramcontent.com/pod-product-compliance
Lightning Source LLC
Chambersburg PA
CBHW050519170426
43201CB00013B/2014